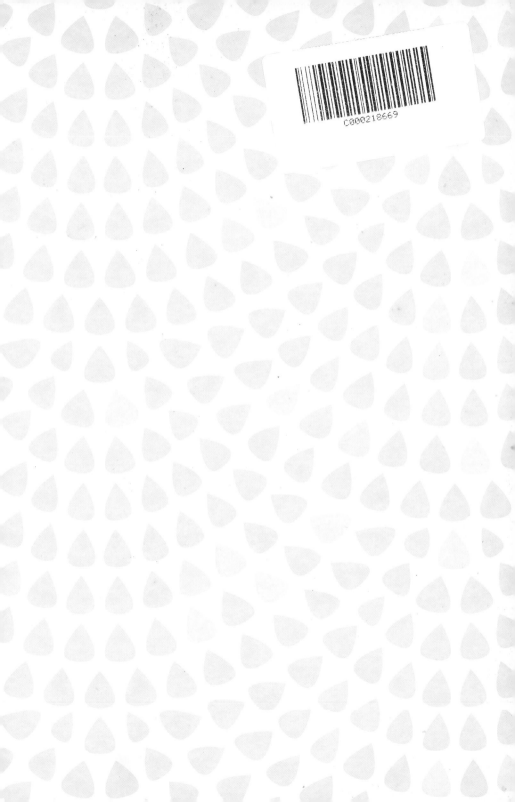

# FRENCH COMPLEXION

Christine Clais (aka the French Facialist) is a French-born skin expert and author renowned for her healing facial treatments and transformative skincare advice. Like most French women, Christine believes that we all have the power to improve our skin by treating it as an integral part of our body, its own ecosystem.

Christine currently lives in Melbourne with her French partner Christophe and their two dogs and cat, Marcel, Lily and Juliette.

www.thefrenchfacialist.com

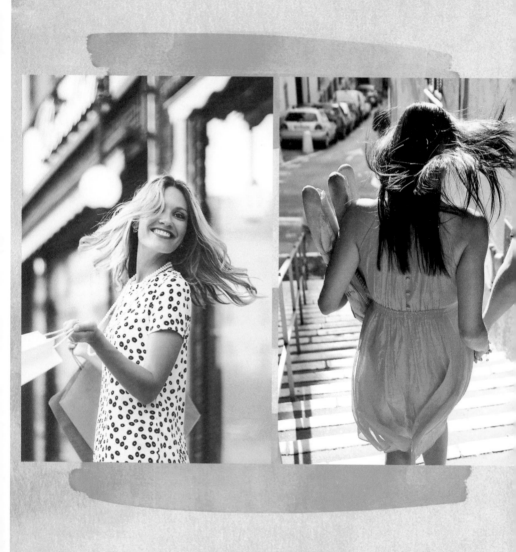

# FRENCH COMPLEXION

## THE SECRETS TO BEAUTIFUL SKIN AT ANY AGE

CHRISTINE CLAIS

VIKING
*an imprint of*
PENGUIN BOOKS

# Contents

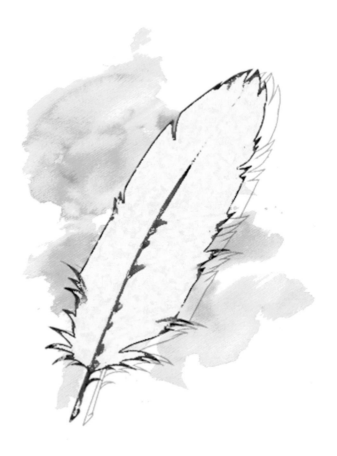

This book is dedicated to Antoine,
my bright light in the sky.

# Manifesto for happy skin

Today, I shall love my skin.

Today, I shall treat my skin with respect and kindness.

Today and every day.

Regardless of where I am or what I am doing.

As my skin hugs and protects me I shall hug and protect my skin back by attending to its needs, my body's needs, my needs.

Nurture

Love

Cherish my skin unconditionally

As an extension of me.

As a part of me.

As me.

Today, I shall love my skin and radiate this love onto my world and the entire universe.

Glow.

*Moi* (me) xx

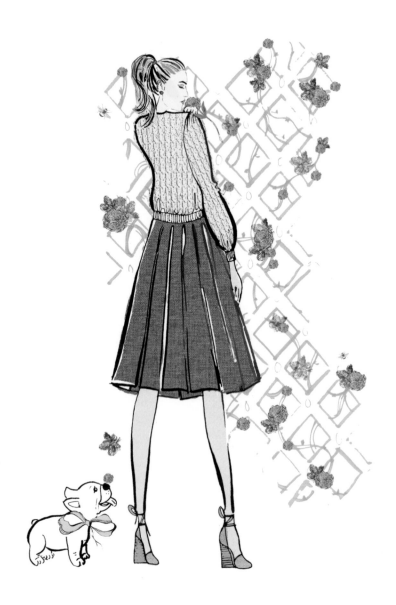

# INTRODUCTION

## MY FRENCH
## SKIN PHILOSOPHY

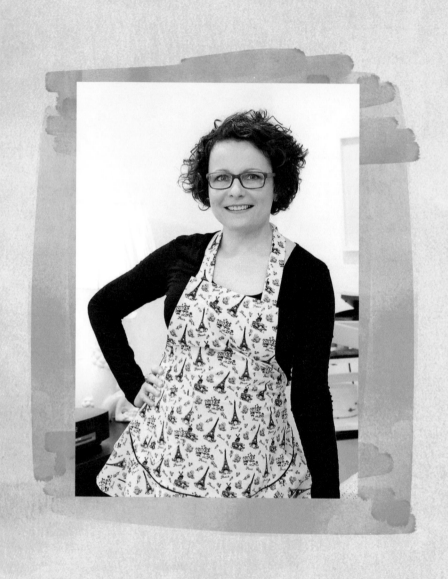

# Bonjour!

My fascination with skin and skincare began as a young girl under the wonderful influence of *Bonne Maman*, my paternal grandmother. I remember *Bonne Maman* telling me about the benefits of using rainwater to cleanse your skin. I have vivid memories of the creams that she used. I was mesmerised by the magic of those pots elegantly displayed in my grandparents' *salle de bain* (bathroom). I can still clearly recall how they looked: light pink and translucent white jars with their luxurious gold lids. Sometimes, I would be allowed to take one home with me. The ultimate treat! To me, it did not matter that they were nearly empty: they were the best presents I could get and I would then try to emulate *Bonne Maman*'s beauty rituals at home.

I also recall my first visit to a beauty salon. It was in Saint-Omer in the north of France, where I grew up. I was fifteen and *Maman*, my loving mother, decided that it was time I experienced my first *nettoyage de peau* (deep cleansing facial), as my skin was going through your typical teenage pimply stage. There I was like a grown-up, proudly lying on a facial bed as the expert hands of Madame Dumont cleansed, exfoliated and massaged my skin. I was sent home with a few products and my skin quickly cleared.

While these early experiences ignited my interest in skincare, it wasn't until I started working as a long-haul flight attendant for Air France (before migrating to Australia twenty-six years ago) that I started to take a more serious interest in facial products and treatments, as I looked for solutions to treat my own very dehydrated, frequent-flying skin. Then, a little over twenty years ago, I decided to study Health Science and become a qualified aesthetician. I have never looked back: I truly found my passion in caring for skin!

I have worked in most settings within the international beauty world: in salons and clinics, in department stores and pharmacies, at fashion events and beauty expos, in training centres and leading spas. These days, I run my own facialist business and I continue to work as the 'hands-on' facialist to my large family of private clients. My treatments are both result-driven and nurturing: I not only address specific skin concerns, I also take care of the entire person whom I have in front of me.

# My French skin philosophy

Like most French women, I have a holistic view of beauty. Holism is a concept that considers a functioning whole to be always more than simply the sum of its individual parts. Viewed in this light, our bodies are ecosystems in which each component (including our skin) interacts with and influences every other component. And, in holistic terms, our lifestyle choices, behaviour, attitudes and emotions – the way we interact with the world – all affect our health and appearance. My own personal life journey as a woman in her fifties, as well as my professional experience as a facialist, have, over time, contributed to the maturing of this conviction: our skin is not only affected by the way we treat it on the surface but also by our general physical and emotional state. And this is why we need to adopt a broad approach to skincare if we want to improve our skin's functioning and appearance.

With this book, my aim is:

1. To share my skincare approach with you: a philosophy based on over twenty years of professional hands-on experience and on the French culture that I have grown up with.
2. To inform you about skin-friendly products, rituals and techniques that can provide true skin healing and skin-ageing management.
3. To encourage you to 'tune in' to your skin's unique characteristics and needs, so you can treat it in the best possible way for YOU.
4. To show you how to obtain and maintain skin that radiates good health and vigour regardless of your age.
5. To foster the concept of feeling good in your skin (or *être bien dans sa peau* as we say in French).

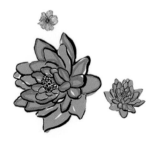

## This book is the right fit for you if:

1. You want to feel confident and happy about the way you look.
2. You are sick of wasting money on ineffective or inadequate skincare products.
3. You crave genuine information based on expert knowledge that has been built on years of hands-on, practical and professional experience.
4. You understand the importance of following a skincare regime but are confused about what to do.
5. You feel overwhelmed by the numerous choices available to you.
6. You want expert skincare advice that is good for your skin, both in the short and long term.
7. You are frightened of invasive cosmetic surgery and intuitively know that it is not for you.
8. You are willing to have an open mind about your skin and life in general.
9. You have always wondered what the secrets are to the apparently effortless beauty that French women seem to possess.

## You might want to give this book a miss if:

1. You believe in a one-dimensional skincare approach that only considers the surface of the skin.
2. You believe that the holy grail of healthy and vibrant skin is to be found in the form of a single 'miracle' product.
3. You believe that cosmetic surgery and injectables can replace looking after yourself and having a consistent skincare regime.

# My skincare approach

I think it is important to remember the true meaning of 'skincare': 'care' for the skin.

I believe that caring for our skin is a life journey of learning and self-discovery. This is why my skincare approach is educational, proactive and empowering. It aims to give you the knowledge necessary for choosing what is best for your skin. It encourages you to listen to the clues that your skin and your entire self give you every day. It emphasises that the most effective skincare choices are the ones that are suited to you. In brief, it allows you to take control of your own skin and to make informed decisions.

I believe that any successful and sustainable attempt at improving the appearance of our skin and delay its ageing should include not only the regular use of suitable skincare products but also, and as importantly, a careful review of our lifestyle choices and the way they can affect our skin.

## This is why my skincare approach is two-fold:
1. *Topical* – using the right combination of products, ingredients and techniques on your skin.
2. *Integrative* – considering your entire self, your general state of health, your wellbeing and your lifestyle.

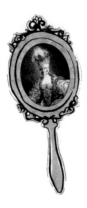

# Beauty secrets of French women

And finally, I must add that the national attitudes and beliefs that I grew up with in France also greatly influence my skincare approach. Despite my years of training in the science of skincare, I find these to be just as important as any beauty product or routine I have ever come across. These are the beauty secrets of French women that I want to convey to you in this book:

## French women believe in an individualistic expression of beauty: 'être soi-même'

French society is dubious of anyone not wanting to look or be like themselves and, in France, being labelled *sans personalité* (with no personality) is the ultimate insult. For this reason, looking like a replica of a celebrity or exactly like your girlfriends is an absolute no-no! French women do use their appearance to showcase their individuality: they might wear the same fashionable items that others are wearing but they will always personalise their outfits by adding a unique vintage or classic touch to them. It might be a belt found at the local *marché aux puces* (trash and treasure market), a unique piece of jewellery, their favourite silk scarf, or some other thing that you will not see on anybody else.

## French women embrace their femininity with understated elegance: 'être féminine'

Looking feminine is important to French women. This does not necessarily mean wearing floral dresses and high heels: it is more of an attitude, a feeling thing! French femininity is expressed in subtle ways and at every age: in the way you stand and walk, in your tone of voice, in the gentle manner in which you display confidence and in all your mannerisms. In France, your femininity is also reflected in the way other people look at you – and people do stare and check you out! In fact, both French women and men are sensitive to beauty and femininity, and they will equally admire the beauty of a 20-year-old or a 70-year-old woman. French women also channel their femininity through the way they view their skin, their body and the ageing process: they are quite at ease with the way they look and quite proud of their appearance too.

### French women like to look natural: *'avoir une apparence naturelle'*

French women do not like to wear heavy make-up as they hate looking *artificiel* (artificial). Rather than hiding or camouflaging their skin, they much prefer to highlight their best features. This more natural look is achieved with the help of some staple items: a tinted moisturiser or lightweight foundation, a touch of blush, some mascara, some lipstick or lip gloss and *voilà*! But of course, this look can only be successfully executed over well-maintained skin. This is why French women take the task of looking after their skin very seriously, NEVER, EVER, compromising their skincare rituals!

### French women follow a regular skincare regime: *'un régime de beauté régulier'*

French women understand the importance of a good home-care regime for their skin. From a very early age, they have seen their grandmothers and mothers unfailingly treating their skin every day and, naturally, they then emulate these home beauty rituals with discipline and rigour.

In France, skincare is taken very seriously and a myriad of high-quality skincare products commonly adorn the shelves and benches of French bathrooms. Indeed, most French women (and increasingly men!) regularly use a cleanser, toner, eye gel or cream, serum, day cream, sunscreen, night cream, exfoliant and mask. And they usually do not stop there: French women are equally into caring for their bodies and regularly use a body scrub, body moisturiser and even bust-firming and anti-cellulite products!

### French women are passionate about everything: *'de la passion dans tout'*

The French are passionate people (*Oui! Je suis passionnée!*). In fact, in France, everything exudes love, romance and passion. This can be a little intense to a non-French person. Let me explain: for example, it is totally normal for French women (and men) to have long and animated discussions on any topic, including relationships, politics and religion. This is not being opinionated or arrogant, this is being passionate and involved! In France, it is also quite acceptable to openly show your feelings and emotions in most situations. In fact, this is expected, this is being passionate. If passion adds zest and beauty to French women's lives, is it a bad thing? Surely not! *J'aime la passion!*

## French women follow a balanced diet: *'un régime alimentaire équilibré'*

French women know that eating well is paramount to looking and remaining youthful for as long as possible. So, cooking a wide variety of fresh and seasonal foods bought at the local market is always the preferred option. Junk food? *Non, merci!*

Everyday meals are composed of small servings and typically include an entrée made of *crudités* (a raw salad), followed by a little meat or fish served with some fresh vegetables of various colours, as well as some lettuce and a little cheese; and perhaps, to finish, a piece of fruit or some yoghurt. Of course, French women like to indulge too, but these culinary excesses are only reserved for special occasions. Champagne, croissants and cakes are special treats and not to be consumed every day.

## French women like walking: *'la marche à pied'*

Although the Gallic nation is more renowned for its champagne and food than for its sporting achievements, French women do like to walk. In fact, walking is so common that it is part of the French lifestyle: you walk to work, you walk to school, you walk to the shops, you go for a long walk with the family on the weekend, you walk everywhere! Walking is definitely seen as the favourite form of exercise by French women: it is not too strenuous, just gentle and effective enough to help you keep healthy and slim. As most French women would say: '*Je n'aime pas la gym, je préfère la marche*', which translates to: 'I do not like going to the gym, I much prefer walking.' Me too!

## French women believe in the power of skin supplementation: *'la dermo-nutrition'*

In France, hundreds of nutritional skin supplements are available for purchase everywhere: in pharmacies, beauty salons and even in mainstream supermarkets like Auchan or Carrefour. In fact, most French skincare houses not only offer traditional skincare products such as cleansers, serums and creams, they also market nutritional capsules, tablets or potions to be consumed in conjunction with their skincare. *L'huile de bourrache* (borage oil) is seen as a favourite for boosting the resilience and integrity of the skin, thanks to its richness in essential fatty acids. A few times a year, French women also love to undergo a herbal detox to help brighten up their skin, reduce fluid retention and increase vitality: all it takes is drinking a daily shot of *complexe drainant aux plantes* (herbal detoxifying elixir) for a week or two. Whatever their supplement selection, French women believe in the synergetic power of a regular skincare regime together with the ingestion of skin food supplements. It is a given!

## French women believe in taking the time to live: '*l'art de vivre*'

In France, people have been resisting the effects of globalisation for a while: for instance, most people oppose the idea of 24-hour or Sunday trading. Why? Because these changes would have too much of a negative impact on their lives. Although this can be frustrating at times to the French expatriate that I am (who is used to the more efficient and fast-paced Anglo-Saxon way of doing things), it is quite endearing to see that French women, regardless of how busy they are, will always make time for what they treat as life essentials: a nutritious three-course lunch with a colleague or a friend, buying fresh food at their local street market, reading a book with a face mask on, or a Sunday walk with the entire family. Their secret lies in resisting the stress of life demands and recognising what is essential to their sense of health and happiness. *L'art de vivre* is all about living in the present moment and appreciating the simplicity of life and what makes you truly happy.

Above all, as you read through this book I would like you to keep in mind that caring for our skin should be enjoyable and empowering. I look forward to supporting you on your journey to skin rejuvenation. As we say in French: *bonne lecture!* (Happy reading!)

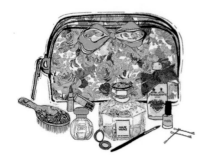

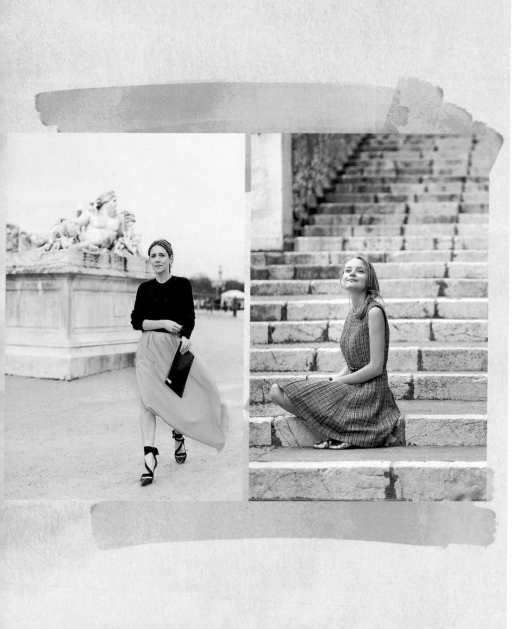

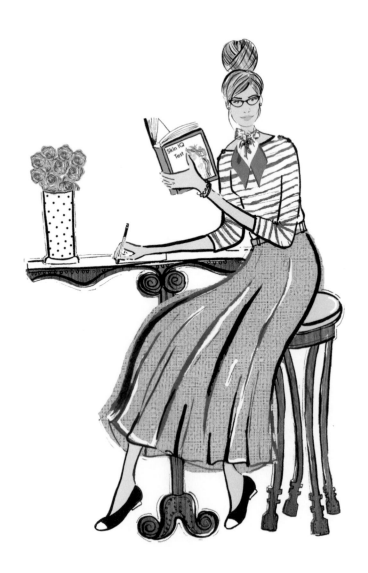

# CHAPTER 1

## GETTING TO KNOW YOUR SKIN

If we're going to look after our skin properly, it helps to know what we are dealing with. So let's first get into the nuts and bolts of what the skin actually is. We probably all know that our skin is our largest organ and that it is made up of various layers, but here is a little more information about it:

# Our skin's three layers

### Epidermis: the layer that we see
The epidermis is the skin's outer layer. New cells are constantly getting produced in its basal layer. As these cells mature, they migrate upwards towards the surface of the skin and eventually die. At the same time, the skin continuously sheds some of its dead surface cells, a process called desquamation.

### Dermis: the layer that houses our precious collagen and elastin fibres
The dermis is the skin's middle layer. It contains our skin's collagen and elastin fibres. Collagen gives the skin its tautness while elastin makes it more elastic. In the dermis, you can also find other important skin components: hair follicles, sebaceous glands, sweat glands, nerves and blood vessels.

### Hypodermis: the layer that supports our skin
The hypodermis is located underneath the dermis. It is mainly composed of fatty tissue, which protects us from sudden changes in temperature and also from physical shock. This cushioning contributes to our skin looking plump and youthful.

- The surface area of our skin covers about 2 square metres.
- Our skin makes up around 16 per cent of our total weight.
- The thickness of our skin ranges from 0.5 millimetres (on our eyelids) to 4 millimetres (on our heels).

(G.J. Tortora & B.H. Derrickson, *Principles of Anatomy and Physiology*, Wiley, New York, 2009, p. 148.)

## Skin facts

Here are some essential skin facts to ponder on:

### Skin fact 1: Our skin is interconnected with the rest of our body

We are often so preoccupied with the appearance of our skin – a pimple, a rash, a wrinkle – that we forget to think of it in terms of a 'living organ'. In fact, our skin is the only one of our organs that we can actually see! More than a mere cover, our skin is an integral part of us, a component that is intrinsically linked to the rest of our body. For instance, our skin works hand in hand with our body's circulatory system since the dermis contains a network of blood vessels that supply our skin with nutrition and oxygen, and also facilitate the elimination of waste products from our body.

### Skin fact 2: Our skin is fundamental to our survival

We need our skin for a variety of reasons: in particular, so it can act as a protective layer against the damage caused by various airborne pollutants and by UV radiation from sunlight; shield us from the risk of infection caused by harmful microbes; and prevent excessive fluid loss from the body. At the same time, our skin is actively involved in thermoregulation (a safety mechanism that ensures that our body temperature remains in a safe range to protect our vital organs) thanks to the action of its sweat glands, among other processes.

## Skin fact 3: Our skin enables us to feel and react to our exterior environment

Our skin helps us detect changes that occur outside of us. Due to its location (the interface between our body and an ever-changing outside world) and also thanks to its network of nerve receptors, our skin allows us to feel the sensations of pressure, touch, pain, cold and heat so we can react to them accordingly. For instance, we usually respond to a gentle massage touch by relaxing, or we have the reflex to quickly lift our hand off a hotplate to avoid a burn.

## Skin fact 4: Our skin can reveal a lot about ourselves

Observing someone's skin can give us some useful clues regarding their health, age or lifestyle choices. It can even help us detect the emotions felt by the person we are looking at: for example, someone can display the feelings of embarrassment or anger through blushing, or show fear by appearing extremely pale or by developing goosebumps. The expression 'to develop a thick skin' illustrates very well the emotional aspect of our largest organ. And so does the French expression '*avoir une sensibilité à fleur de peau*' which literally translates as 'to have a sensitivity close to the skin' – meaning to be hypersensitive.

Let's now find out some specifics about your unique skin:

# Classifying your skin

As you might not always be in a position to get some skincare advice from a professional, or you might simply prefer to select your skincare yourself, it does help to know the basics of skin analysis. No need to get into complicated diagnostics here. There are just three main questions relating to your skin that you should answer before you go shopping for new products. Getting your answers right is crucial, as failing to correctly identify your skin type and the condition it is in usually leads to choosing the wrong products and worsening your skin's condition. This is especially important when selecting your facial cleanser and moisturiser – the two products that constitute the backbone of a good skincare regime.

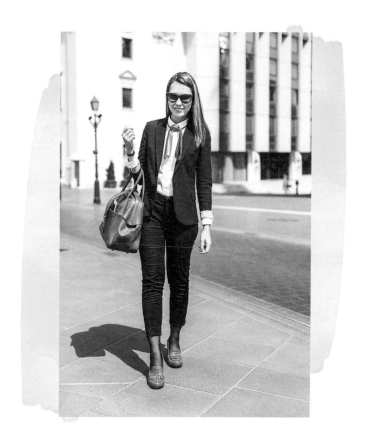

## Step 1: Is your skin oily, normal, dry or combination?

This question relates to your skin's oil content, which is highly influenced by your genes and your hormones. Look for the following signs, which will give you an indication of where your skin is on the oily-to-dry skin spectrum, 'normal' being at the middle:

*Characteristics of oily skin:*

- Can appear shiny (but not always).
- Enlarged pores are commonly seen.
- Blackheads are usually found.
- Whiteheads may be present.
- Breakouts (pimples) are common.
- Acne may be present.

A blackhead (or open comedone) is a mixture of dead skin cells and hardened sebum that obstructs the opening of a hair follicle (pore), preventing the natural elimination of oil and cell debris from the follicle. Its surface looks black because it has oxidised once in contact with the air.

A whitehead (or closed comedone) is similar in composition to a blackhead. However, it is less noticeable because of the fact that it does not cause the hair follicle opening to fully dilate, which also means that the oxidation process cannot occur.

A pimple can be classified into either a 'papule' or a 'pustule' and indicates that inflammation is present in the skin. A pimple first appears as a papule (a small, red and usually sore pimple). When enough infection-fighting white blood cells have raised to the surface of the skin, this papule may then develop into a pustule (a pimple with pus showing on top).

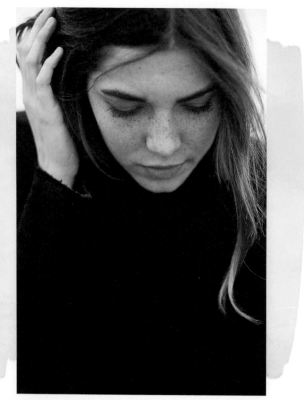

*Characteristics of normal skin:*
- Looks plump and radiant.
- Has a smooth texture.
- Shows no sign of enlarged pores.
- Shows no sign of congestion.
- Breakouts (pimples) are uncommon.

*Characteristics of dry skin:*
- Can look dry and flaky.
- Fine lines and wrinkles can be apparent.
- Can feel itchy, tight and rough.
- Enlarged pores are not commonly seen.*
- Shows no sign of congestion.
- Breakouts (pimples) are extremely uncommon.
- Eczema and dermatitis may be present. Can easily become sensitised (see step 3).

* Please note that if enlarged pores are present on dry skin, they indicate that skin was oily in younger years.

*Combination skin:*

It is not uncommon to have skin that shows different skin types in various areas of the face. Indeed, most people have an oilier T-zone while the rest of the face is normal or dry. The presence of different skin types on the face is commonly referred to as 'combination skin'.

The T-zone is the area of facial skin that covers the forehead, the nose and the chin, in the shape of the letter T, hence its name.

## Step 2: Is your skin dehydrated?

Dehydrated skin can show similarities with dry skin. Both can look lined and flaky, and both can feel tight and rough to the touch. However, the two should not be confused since skin 'dryness' relates to a lack of oil and 'dehydration' refers to a lack of moisture in the skin. While the level of water in the epidermis is closely linked to its oil content (dry skin is more likely to be dehydrated than oily skin), it is totally possible for oily skin to be dehydrated too. In fact, the skin of most people that I see, regardless of their skin type, shows some degree of dehydration. This lack of moisture can be caused by a myriad of reasons, the main ones being an irregular skincare regime, using the wrong products for one's skin or in the wrong way, living in a dry climate, and various lifestyle factors.

*WARNING: Misdiagnosing your oily but dehydrated skin for dry skin is likely to lead you to use products that are too heavy for your skin, which in turn will exacerbate your skin congestion and/or breakouts.*

———————

*Characteristics of oily + dehydrated skin:*
- Can appear shiny (but not always).
- Enlarged pores are commonly seen.
- Blackheads are usually found.
- Whiteheads may be present.
- Breakouts (pimples) are common.
- Acne may be present.
- Fine lines may be seen.
- Can be flaky.
- Can feel tight.
- Can have a rough texture (localised or all over).

## Step 3: Is your skin currently sensitised?

I find that a lot of people are quick to self-diagnose their skin as being 'sensitive' when it is, in fact, 'sensitised'. Let me explain the difference: you may have skin that is delicate and reactive by nature: 'sensitive' skin (like my own skin!). But having sensitive skin is not a problem per se if your skin is also healthy and well balanced (and, therefore, unlikely to react adversely). On the other hand, you would classify your skin as being 'sensitised' if it were currently causing you a high level of sensitivity, regardless of its general type.

The fact is that anyone's skin, even the thickest and most resilient, can go through times of heightened sensitivity and become sensitised by a variety of factors including general life stresses, ill-health, harsh climate conditions, poor lifestyle and the wrong skincare choices (this includes doing too much to your skin!). Note that you do not need to experience all of these stressors at once in order to develop skin sensitisation: a single one can set your skin off.

*Characteristics of sensitised skin:*

- Is more sensitive than usual.
- Can look red.
- Can look inflamed.
- Can feel hot.
- Can feel tight.
- Can feel sensitive and 'achy'.
- Can sting and burn.
- Can look aged.
- Can look flaky.
- May have a rough texture.
- Can be intolerant of skincare products.

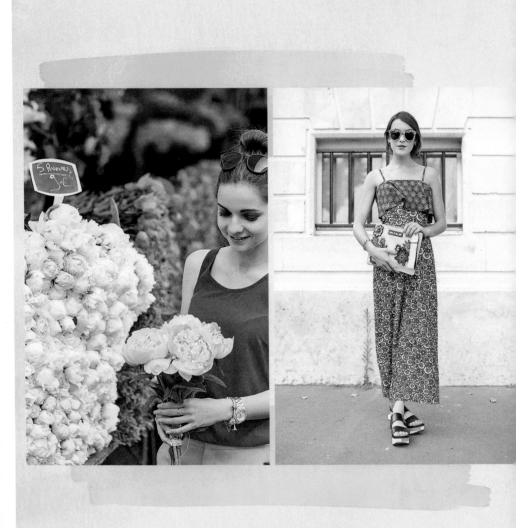

# Understanding the ageing process of our skin

When I ask my new clients what their main skin concerns are, ageing usually tops the list. Indeed, I find that most women I meet want to know how to look younger and how to delay the ageing process of their skin as much as possible. The first step in looking more youthful is to understand the various reasons why our skin ages.

## Getting older

Like the rest of our body, our skin is destined to age; it is a fact! This natural ageing process is determined by our genes, which control our lifespan. It is also influenced by changes in our hormone levels as we reach puberty, middle age and beyond. And as life goes by, our skin becomes drier and thinner, starts to lose its plumpness and develops lines and wrinkles.

*Accepting the natural cycle of life wholeheartedly is the only way to age well and be happy! But this does not mean that we should have a fatalistic attitude towards ageing, as there are many ways to assist the skin so it can mature well and be radiant at any age.*

*Let's rejoice in the fact that the worst visible signs of ageing are caused by factors that we can easily control: notably, our exposure to free radicals and our poor skincare habits.*

## The damaging action of free radicals

Free radicals can cause havoc in our skin. These are highly unstable chemical substances that can latch onto our skin components and have a detrimental effect on them. For instance, they have the power to damage our DNA, to denature our collagen and elastin fibres (which are paramount to our skin looking young), and they are also able to reduce our skin's ability to repair itself. In his book *The Wrinkle Cure*, Nicholas Perricone, MD, colourfully describes the action of free radicals: 'Unfortunately, much like an out-of-control guy in a singles bar, free radicals get into lots of unhealthy relationships and do their unsuspecting partners – other molecules and atoms – a good deal of harm.' (N. Perricone, *The Wrinkle Cure*, Warner Books, New York, 2000, p. 48.)

The sheer fact of being alive causes the formation of free radicals, as by-products of our metabolism. Although our bodies possess built-in mechanisms to neutralise these bad guys, their fighting powers are limited and they cannot cope with the entire excess of free radicals that are produced by our lifestyle factors (such as stress, smoking, pollution, poor dietary choices or overexposure to UV radiation from the sun).

## Our poor skincare habits

What we do (or do not do) to our skin can also significantly contribute to its premature ageing. Indeed, over-treating or under-treating our skin, and using products that are too harsh or drying, can contribute to a weakening of its vital barrier function and make it more susceptible to inflammation and ageing.

In my opinion, the fashionable overuse of potent cosmeceutical skincare products is currently contributing to the emergence of a generation of women with stripped, sensitised and damaged skin that will not age well if they continue to treat it so harshly for too long (more on cosmeceuticals in Chapter 2).

*Say 'NON' to self-induced skin damage and ageing caused by overexposure to free radicals and poor skincare habits. ALWAYS treat your skin and yourself with kindness!*

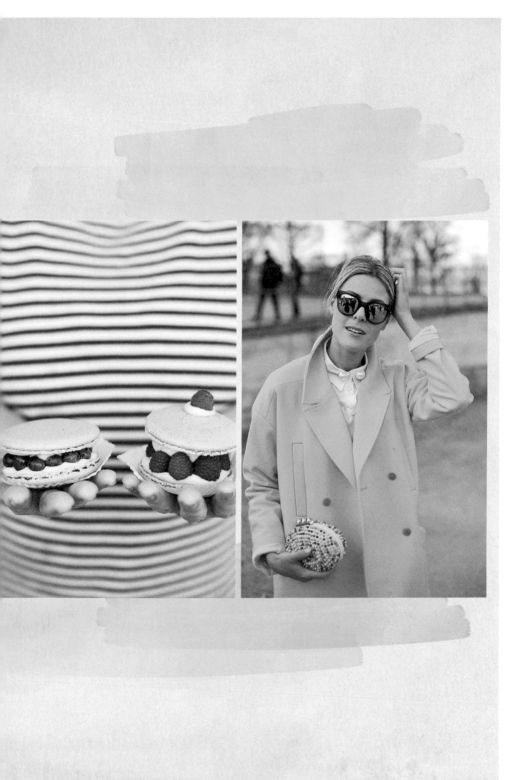

# Embracing ageing like a French woman

Since we are now living longer, sixty seems to have become the new forty everywhere! But one point that I need to express here is that, as a whole, French society appears to be much kinder to older women than most other nations are.

In fact, it is totally okay to be a mature woman in France since the French will always admire your natural beauty and your elegance regardless of your age.

What matters the most to my compatriots is to be well-groomed and well-mannered. (And yes, the French can be quite critical of anyone who *n'a pas la classe* – does not have class – and who does not try to spruce up!)

As a mature French woman myself, I am lucky to have countless examples of older female role models who are absolutely revered in my own country:

* Juliette Binoche, 52 (actress, dancer and human rights campaigner)
* Jane Birkin, 69 (actress, singer and ex-partner of the late Serge Gainsbourg)
* Rachida Dati, 50 (former French Minister of Justice and current member of the European Parliament)
* Catherine Deneuve, 72 (actress and film producer)
* Inès de la Fressange, 58 (model and fashion designer)
* Isabelle Huppert, 63 (actress)
* Christine Lagarde, 60 (lawyer, former French Minister of Finance and current head of the IMF)
* Jeanne Moreau, 88 (actress, screenwriter and film director)
* Kristin Scott Thomas, 55 (actress)
* Simone Veil, 88 (lawyer and politician)

and many many more!

All these iconic women have their own personal style and all look *naturelles* (natural), which is partly why they are so well-respected.

(Oh, and I would like to add Françoise Clais, 87, to the list: my mother, the most talented seamstress in the world, handywoman extraordinaire, an avid reader of French history books, with a no-nonsense and honest approach to life and so much generosity of spirit. *Merci Maman* for being such an excellent role model!)

*When you exude personality, inner strength and self-acceptance, people are more likely to respect you since your self-image is not so dependent on the opinion of others. So, let's do what the French do: let's not obsess about ageing and let's focus more on nurturing ourselves and our skin. YES, we can all be self-confident and happy at any age!*

## My views on cosmetic surgery and injectables

Personally, I am not a fan of cosmetic surgery procedures. I prefer enhancing my natural features via the self-care habits that I describe in this book. This way I not only take care of my skin's daily needs but also my entire being's needs. I simply find this approach much more self-empowering.

As a professional facialist, I believe that cosmetic work SHOULD NEVER be considered as a skincare approach but rather as a last resort when everything else has failed to make you love the way you look.

I have countless clients who were seriously considering getting jabbed by a needle before they first started seeing me: they felt old and rugged and they wanted to look younger. But by committing to my skincare approach, they were not only able to improve their skin but also change the way they viewed themselves, thus eliminating or delaying the compulsion to visit a cosmetic clinic.

I also have a serious issue with some doctors recommending anti-wrinkle injections to young women as a preventative measure against developing wrinkles. Duty of care, perhaps? @#%&@#! Pardon my French!

*Since we all have the power to transform our skin, why not take control by making some positive skincare, lifestyle and mindset changes?*

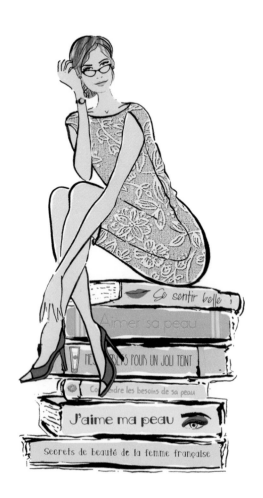

# CHAPTER 2

## THE IMPORTANCE OF
## SKINCARE
## RITUALS

# French women's time-tested skincare rituals

A lot has been written about French women, most of which tends to be terribly cliché and make most non-French women feel slightly unworthy or inadequate. But let me reassure you here: as both a French woman and an experienced facialist, I can certify that, regardless of where we women come from, we all have insecurities and fears. We all have good days and bad days, we all want to look and feel the best we can. And we all need to work at feeling good and loving ourselves. French women as much as any other women. Full stop.

But one strong resource French women can always rely on is their deep-rooted skincare rituals; those good, time-tested habits that were instilled in them at a very young age.

Indeed, as a young French girl, you are taught to care for your skin in the same way you are shown how to care for your teeth or the rest of your body. You are given good and sound skincare advice by your mother, grandmother and every other woman around you! So, you take it all as a given and you go on emulating these skincare steps throughout your life. Not a bad thing at all, considering that our skin responds so well to rituals.

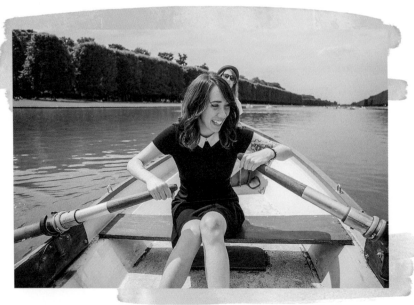

# Our skin responds well to rituals

Our skin needs looking after. In fact, it requires a minimum level of daily attention and care to ensure its protection and assist its proper functioning.

*We do not need to spend hours on our skin to get noticeable results but sticking to an everyday routine is the key to helping keep our skin healthy, improve our complexion and make us look more youthful.*

Developing and maintaining daily skincare habits is the essence here: no matter how good your skincare products are, you will never get the best out of them unless you use them regularly. I hear you: 'Easier said than done!' Life does get so busy sometimes that it can be a real challenge to find time for yourself and your skin. Long hours at work, the arrival of a new baby, looking after elderly parents, starting a new business, etc. . . . Caring for your skin is often the first thing to go.

So, how can you keep up good skincare habits when your life gets out of control?

The answer is to simplify your daily routine to the basics so it only takes a few minutes a day (6 minutes!). This way, your skin still benefits, and your skincare regime is more likely to feel like a quick self-nurturing 'me time' rather than another chore added to your exhaustive (and exhausting) list of daily tasks.

**EXPERT TIP**

In the evening, cleanse and moisturise your skin as soon as you get home, to eliminate the risk of not doing it because you feel too tired later on!

# The 6-minute daily facial skincare routine

## Morning

Step 1: Cleanse face, neck and décolletage (60 seconds max).

Step 2: Apply eye gel/cream to the eye contour area (30 seconds max).

Step 3: Apply face cream/sunscreen to face, neck and décolletage (90 seconds max).

## Evening

Step 1: Cleanse face, neck and décolletage (90 seconds max).

Step 2: Apply eye gel/cream to the eye contour area (30 seconds max).

Step 3: Apply face cream to face, neck and décolletage (60 seconds max).

> Did you know...?
>
> *Décolletage* (or *décolleté*) is a French word that describes the neckline that you show when you wear a low-cut top or dress.

# A little more

Once you have mastered the basics of skincare, consider adding a little more to your skincare regime. Here is what you need to do to complete your skincare rituals:

## Additional daily step (once or twice a day):

- Use a serum to treat specific skin concerns. A serum can be applied either all over your face, neck and décolletage or on defined areas only, depending on where your skin concerns are. (See more information on serums in Chapter 4.)

## Additional weekly steps (once or twice a week):

- Exfoliate your face, neck and décolletage.
- Use a facial mask on your face, neck and décolletage.

These extra steps might add 20 to 30 minutes to your total weekly skincare rituals, but they will take your skin to the next level of radiance. They are totally worth this extra time!

## THE GOLDEN RULES OF SKINCARE RITUALS

1. You do need to stick to a routine: every day, morning and night.
2. It is essential that the skincare products you use are perfectly suited to you.
3. Everything that you do to your skin should be with a loving and caring intent.

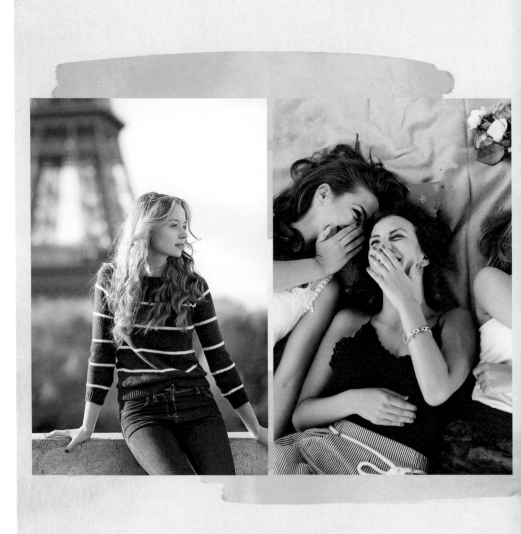

# At what age should we start using skincare products?

Like my French compatriots, I believe that a skincare routine should be established early so it becomes second nature to you.

All French kids would have had their first taste of skincare as toddlers since French mothers are very big on sun protection for their children and themselves. I do remember my own mother regularly chasing my brother and me when we were little so she could re-apply sunscreen on our pale skin during our summer holidays spent in Juan-les-Pins near Cannes in the South of France!

By the time they have reached the age of six to eight, most French girls are already following a simplified skincare regime consisting of cleansing and moisturising their face. They copy their mums' beauty routines with enthusiasm and pride, using cleansing milks and moisturisers from ranges such as La Roche-Posay, Mustela, Avène or Nuxe, products that were purchased especially for them at the local pharmacy or supermarket. The French beauty routine expands to its full amplitude at puberty (or the time at which you start getting the odd blemish) and once it is established, it is to last for the rest of your life. These complete skincare rituals include all essential and advanced skincare steps as described in this book.

*If you have not established regular skincare habits yet, start now! And don't worry, it is never too late to care for your skin!*

# Using the right products for your skin

Often, in my work, I am introduced to new clients who have been using the wrong products for their particular skin type (or using them in the wrong way) and, as a result, have unwittingly caused damage to their skin. Keep in mind that because a particular cleanser or cream suited your skin two years ago, this does not mean that it is still is the best one for you! The same goes for the opinions of your girlfriends or your favourite beauty blogger: the fact that they rave about their 'hero' skincare products does not necessarily make these products the ideal choice for you. Instead:

- **See 'Classifying your skin' in Chapter 1.** This should help you determine what kind of skin you have and help you select the right skincare for you.

- **If you are still not sure about your current skin type and condition, why not consult with a facialist who can perform a thorough analysis of your complexion?** To get the most out of your session, it is always a good idea to bring along with you all the skincare products that you have been using (including make-up items), so that your skin expert has a clear understanding of what might be affecting your skin's current appearance and condition.

- **Always keep in mind that it is important to adjust your skincare products in accordance with your skin's changing needs.** Your skin not only goes through changes with age, it is also affected by the seasons, your lifestyle, your stress levels and your general state of health. Hence the need to constantly reassess your skin.

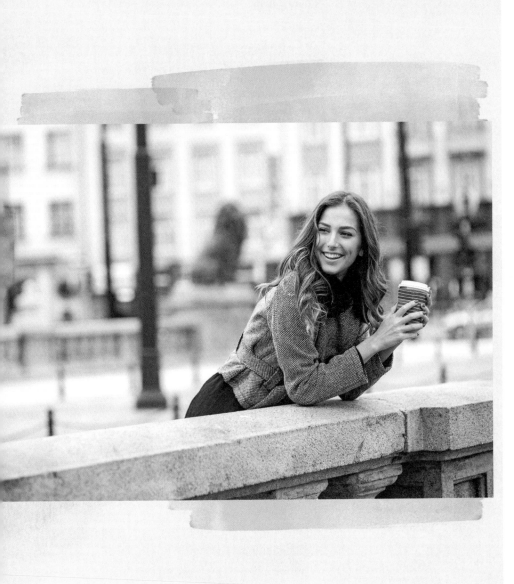

# General skincare guidelines

- **Strengthening your skin and bringing it back to a healthier state should be your primary goal.** While your skin may be currently sensitised and reactive to what you put on it, that is not to say that you cannot strengthen it: as your skin is a living organ, it changes all the time. This means that you can improve it and make it more resilient by reinforcing its barrier function.

- **Act straight away: this means reviewing your state of health, lifestyle and current skincare regime to try and identify your sensitising triggers.** Sometimes, this can feel a bit like detective work but if you tune in and pay attention to the way your skin responds to certain things in your life, you will find the culprit(s)! Is it a skincare product? A sensitivity to some foods? Stress? Emotions? A reaction to some medication? Obviously, once you have found your triggers, you must then work at eliminating them in order for your skin to improve.

- **Regardless of what may have caused your skin to become sensitised, you must temporarily alter your current skincare regime until your skin gets better.** If you use products that are too harsh or too active on your weakened complexion, or if you overstimulate it by using too many products or by treating your skin roughly, you are likely to amplify your skin's symptoms of strain and reach a crisis point.

- **Use products that are low-scented or free of added fragrance.** Look for the term 'hypoallergenic' on the packaging, which means that the product is less likely to create an adverse skin reaction. An example of a good range that is specifically designed for sensitised skin is the **La Roche-Posay Toleriane range.**

- **Adopt a simple routine with a minimum amount of products and focus on gently cleansing and moisturising your skin, and nothing else, until your skin improves.** This could take a few weeks to a few months, depending on the severity of your symptoms. Remember that 'less is more' until your skin picks up.

- **As your skin improves, start introducing other steps to your skincare routine.** Slowly incorporate other products such as a gentle exfoliant and a soothing or hydrating mask.
- **Wait until all signs of skin trauma have disappeared to resume a complete routine.** You can then start supercharging your skincare routine with products targeting your specific concerns (such as oiliness, congestion, breakouts including acne, pigmentation, ageing, etc.).

## If you have either normal, oily or dry skin

- **If your skin is normal, make sure to do everything in your power to keep it this way as long as possible.** Your normal skin is unlikely to cause you any concerns, which is fabulous. But do not take your skin for granted as it can still get damaged and become sensitised if forgotten about or treated harshly. Never get tempted to adopt a nonchalant attitude towards skincare!
- **If your skin is oily, it is likely to drive you crazy.** Shiny, congested, prone to breaking out or even going through a serious acne stage . . . Do not despair: your skin does not have to be a source of stress since its oiliness can be controlled by a regular skincare regime. Make sure to adopt the full skincare routine (that also includes using a serum, an exfoliant and a mask), and to read Chapter 5 for useful tips on dealing with your skin problems.
- **If your skin is dry, your main aim will be to keep it nourished at all times.** Those good fats and oils, this is what your skin needs to age well. Oh, and do not forget to exfoliate your skin weekly to get the best out of these rich products: less dead skin-cell build-up on the surface means better product penetration and results.
- **Make sure to respond to your skin's changing needs.** Having a distinct skin type does not mean that it will remain the same all your life. Always remember that your skin is in a constant state of change regardless of its type. For instance, as skin tends to become drier as we age, the oily skin that you had in your twenties could well be quite

normal now that you are older (you might still notice some open pores but your sebaceous glands would now be producing much less oil than before). The same applies for normal skin that is likely to become dry with age, and for naturally dry skin that will always become even drier as time goes by.

### If you have combination skin

- **Choose your cleanser in accordance with the skin type outside your T-zone.** For instance, if your T-zone is oily but the rest of your face is on the normal or drier side, choose a cleanser for either normal skin or all skin types. This way, you will avoid drying out your skin.
- **If your facial skin types are not diametrically opposed, use a moisturiser for normal or combination skin.** If need be, you can also use a serum for oily skin on the most oily part of your face (usually the T-zone) underneath your moisturiser, or a hydrating serum on the drier part (usually the cheeks) underneath your moisturiser. (This latter solution works well for me. Although I have mature skin, my skin still has a decent level of oil which means that I tend to get the odd spot if I use a cream that is too heavy for my T-zone.)
- **If your facial skin types are diametrically opposed, you can use two different moisturisers on your face.** For example, you may have really dry skin on the forehead and cheeks, together with a very oily nose and chin that are prone to blackheads and breakouts. In this case, it may be best to use two creams to suit each of your distinct skin types: one cream for dry skin and another for a more oily skin type.
- **You can also adapt the application technique of your moisturiser to better suit your skin's needs.** To do this, apply more cream on the driest areas of your skin first and finish with a very light application of cream where your skin is at its oiliest.

## If you have dehydrated + oily skin

- **First and foremost, remember that oily skin must never be overfed.** Dehydrated, oily skin needs water, not oil! Use a light-textured, water-based cream. If need be, you can also use a serum for oily skin on the most oily part of your face (usually the T-zone) before the cream.
- **At the same time, avoid using harsh cleansing products.** This would only worsen the dehydration. And when your skin becomes deeply dehydrated, it loses it suppleness and tends to become more congested and more prone to breakouts. Instead, go for a gentle cleansing wash marketed for all skin types.
- **Get right into facial masking!** In order to treat both skin concerns, alternate between a purifying mask and one that has hydrating properties.
- **Purchase an Evian or La Roche-Posay mineral water spray.** Use your spray after cleansing, over your moisturiser or your make-up. Carry it with you and spritz anywhere, anytime!

## If you have dehydrated + dry skin

- **Use both hydrating and nourishing products on your skin: it will loooove them all!** Be partial to cleansing oils and cleansing creams, hy-drating serums, rich moisturisers, facial oils, hydrating and nourishing masks . . . any product that has the words 'hydrating' and 'nourishing' on it!
- **Don't forget to use a facial exfoliant.** You will get better results from your hydrating and nourishing products after you have exfoliated: you need to get rid of the accumulation of dead skin cells that are sitting the surface of your skin first!
- **Invest in a good quality nourishing cream. Gernetic Cytobi** would have to be the one! See 'Moisturising your skin' and my other product recommendations in Chapter 3.

# Cosmeceuticals: c'est quoi?

'Cosmeceutical' would have to be THE beauty buzzword *du jour*. This term, coined about 30 years ago by American dermatologist Albert Kligman, comes from the merging of two words: COSMEtics and pharmaCEUTICAL. It hints at the potency of a particular type of cosmetic products with skin-correcting and 'anti-ageing' ingredients.

Cosmeceutical ranges look like any other skincare ranges but their brand name is usually followed by the word 'cosmeceuticals', which indicates that the focus of the brand is on 'correcting' the skin rather than just hydrating or nourishing it.

This type of skincare usually contains active ingredients such as vitamin C, hyaluronic acid, peptides, stem cells, fruit acids (AHAs or BHAs) and retinol (vitamin A). Even though any skincare brand (cosmeceutical or not) can include these active ingredients, cosmeceutical ranges tend to contain them in much higher concentrations, which usually makes them more potent and more effective at treating skin problems and reducing the visible signs of ageing.

## Key corrective active ingredients

### Vitamin C

Vitamin C is known to encourage the formation of collagen in the skin. Other useful effects of vitamin C are its strengthening action on blood capillaries (it can be recommended for people with a tendency to dilated capillaries and redness) and also its lightening effect on the skin (it is found in a lot of skin 'whitening' products).

### PRECAUTIONS

DO NOT use vitamin C if you are (or recently were) on Roaccutane, as this drug would have thinned, dried out and sensitised your skin. ALWAYS consult with your doctor first.

Topical application of vitamin C can cause skin irritation, especially if your skin is not used to this ingredient. In order to avoid this effect, it is best to introduce it slowly.

If you are unsure on how and when to use it, seek personalised advice from your skincare specialist.

## Retinol (vitamin A)

Retinol has many benefits in terms of improving the appearance of skin. Since it promotes cell renewal and stimulates collagen production, it can effectively smooth lines and wrinkles, refine open pores and even out pigmentation. It can also assist in the treatment of acne by helping to eliminate skin congestion and preventing breakouts.

### PRECAUTIONS

DO NOT use vitamin A products if you are planning to become pregnant, are pregnant, or are breastfeeding.

DO NOT use vitamin A if you are (or recently were) on Roaccutane, as this drug would have thinned, dried out and sensitised your skin. ALWAYS consult with your doctor first.

Since vitamin A can make your skin sensitive to sunlight, it is best to: use at night time; avoid sun exposure; and wear a broad-spectrum, high-factor sunscreen during the day. You may also want to avoid using it during the summer months.

Common side effects include dryness and peeling, irritation and discomfort. In order to minimise these, it is best to introduce it slowly to your skin and to seek advice from your doctor or skincare specialist.

Always follow the manufacturer's instructions.

If you are unsure on how and when to use it, seek personalised advice from your skincare specialist.

## Alpha hydroxy acids (AHAs)

The most well-known AHAs are glycolic acid and lactic acid. These fruit acids have good exfoliating properties which make them particularly helpful for the treatment of aged and sun-damaged skin. Glycolic and lactic acids can help reduce the depth of wrinkles, lighten dark pigmentation spots and boost skin hydration levels. They are known to stimulate collagen production and may also be beneficial when treating acne.

### PRECAUTIONS

DO NOT use AHAs if you are (or recently were) on Roaccutane, as this drug would have thinned, dried out and sensitised your skin. ALWAYS consult with your doctor first.

AHA products can increase your skin's sensitivity to the sun. This is why it is best to use them at night and also to protect your skin with sunscreen during the day.

If you are unsure on how and when to use them, seek personalised advice from your skincare specialist.

## Beta hydroxy acids (BHAs)

The most widely used BHA, salicylic acid, is great to use on oilier skin types or on acne.

DO NOT use BHAs if you are (or recently were) on Roaccutane, as this drug would have thinned, dried out and sensitised your skin. ALWAYS consult with your doctor first.

If you are trying to become pregnant, are pregnant or are breastfeeding, consult your doctor prior to using them.

BHA products can increase your skin's sensitivity to the sun. This is why it is best to use them at night and also to protect your skin with sunscreen during the day.

Do not use salicylic acid if you are allergic to aspirin, as it is derived from the same active ingredient as aspirin.

If you are unsure on how and when to use them, seek personalised advice from your skincare specialist.

## WARNING: beware of the power of cosmeceutical skincare!

Don't get me wrong, I really like cosmeceutical products. In fact, I do use them on my skin, and I do prescribe them to my clients when appropriate. But I am extremely alarmed by the amount of skin damage caused by their overuse. In the last couple of years I have noticed a dramatic increase in the number of clients with extremely sensitised, irritated or damaged skin. And every week, I see at least one or two new clients wanting me to fix their sensitised, raw-looking skin that has resulted from an overload of corrective ingredients that are often hidden in cosmeceutical products.

*BEWARE: an overuse of cosmeceutical products can lead to a weakening of the barrier function of your skin, which in turn causes dehydration, skin irritation and eventual skin damage and premature ageing.*

## Points to remember when using corrective ingredients

1. It is advisable to consult a skincare professional for advice before embarking on a new skincare regime that includes products that contain any of the previously mentioned corrective active ingredients.

2. Introduce these ingredients to your skin with caution. The 'less is more' rule is always best to start with: fewer products, in smaller amounts, left on the skin for a shorter amount of time, and used less often.

3. Always follow manufacturer's instructions.

4. Make sure to keep your skin well hydrated by also incorporating good moisturising products into your skincare regime.

5. Monitor your skin for signs of dehydration and sensitisation (see my general skincare guidelines in the previous part of this chapter) and ease off or discontinue using if your skin starts to look depleted or irritated. No need to strip your skin right down to the bone!

6. Please, do not adhere to the false belief that you will get better results by fanatically using strong products all the time: this philosophy is damaging to the skin.

*Do what French women do: their skincare priority is always to keep their skin well-moisturised and nourished. This, for me, is the best skincare approach if you want to age well: gentle, consistent and nurturing. No stripping the skin's natural barrier, no inflammation and no trauma!*

# My guidelines to consider before buying new skin-care

- **Beware of brands that promise miracle results in an instant.** The skin is an organ that has its own rhythm of regeneration: the epidermis renews itself every twenty-eight days and even longer when we are older. So, any product will need some time to show its real effect on the skin.
- **Always remember that pretty packaging does not ensure the performance of a product.** What is truly important is what is in it! This is why I recommend that you familiarise yourself with the most common skincare active ingredients and their action on the skin.
- **Looking at the ingredient listing will also help you determine the concentration of active ingredients in a skincare product:** the closer an ingredient is to the top of the list, the greater its proportion in the product and the more active it is.
- **A higher price tag does not always guarantee the superiority of a product, but it can indicate a higher product quality and strength.** 'Professional' skincare brands (the ones used by professional facialists) tend to be more expensive than the ones that you see at the supermarket because they usually contain more active ingredients, which means that they are more likely to make a noticeable difference to your skin.
- **Low-scented or fragrance-free products are less likely to cause skin irritations and allergic reactions than strongly scented ones.** This is a fact that you should keep in mind especially if you have naturally sensitive and reactive skin, or if your skin is currently sensitised.
- **Do not believe everything you are told, and test the knowledge of your skincare professional by asking lots of questions.** This way, you should be able to judge her/his level of care, expertise and commitment to helping you choose the right products for you.

Which skincare brand should you select?

I always tell my clients that I do not care about brand names but that I prefer to consider skincare products for the ingredients they contain and for their specific actions on the skin. Of course, looking at a brand name can give you an indication of the source of your products, the manufacturer's level of dedication to research and development, as well as the points of difference of the company in regard to its formulations (botanical, marine-based, using specific active ingredients, natural, etc. . . . ). But selecting your skincare products based on the marketing hype of a particular brand is not wise, as it does not guarantee the quality and efficacy of a skincare program. You usually have to pick products from several brands to find the perfect routine that works for your skin. But of course, this is not usually what skincare companies will tell you as they would rather you spend all of your cosmetic budget on their one brand!

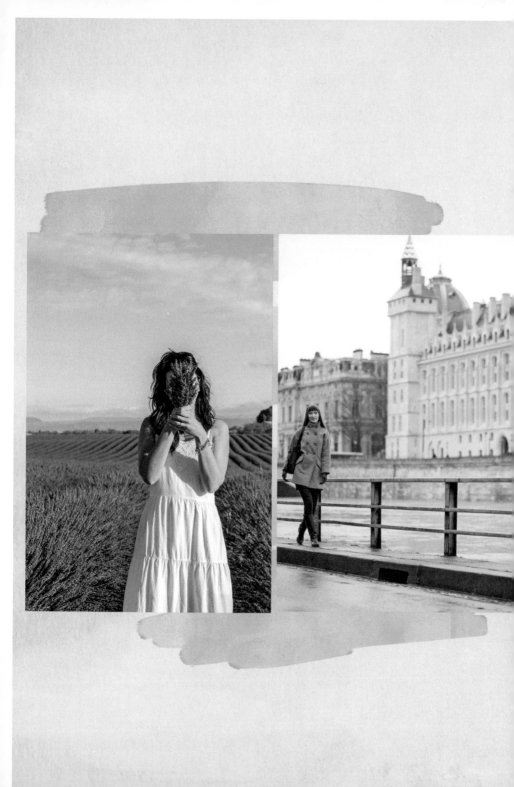

## 'Red flags' to look for when talking to a skincare specialist

Shopping for new skincare can be a fun experience but it can also sometimes be a bit daunting, especially if you are not happy with the current state of your skin. Regardless of where you go (department store, pharmacy, concept store, spa, beauty salon or clinic), you should expect nothing less than great service. Watch for the following warning signs that could indicate that you might be better off going elsewhere:

### 1. You are not given privacy

The information shared during a skincare consultation should be treated as private and confidential, so no one else should be able to hear the conversation that is taking place between you and your skincare specialist. For this reason, you should be given access to a quiet and private area where you can feel comfortable and relaxed.

### 2. You are made to feel rushed

Selecting new skincare products can take a little time and it is usually not done well if conducted in a hurry. In order to make the right choice, your skincare professional should take you through a thorough consultation during which you have the chance to talk about your skin. You should also be given the opportunity to ask any questions that might help you make the best-informed decision about your skin.

### 3. You are not being asked systematic questions

A proper and methodical skincare consultation should cover all areas that could be playing a part in your skin's current state. These include your past and present medical state (so as to avoid contraindicated skincare ingredients) and your lifestyle, as well as your current (and sometimes past) skincare regime. Answers to these questions will constitute the framework for the design of a good skincare regime.

## 4. You are not being asked about your skin concerns

You should be asked clearly about your skin concerns so they can be adequately identified and addressed. Your uppermost skin concern might be different from the one your skincare specialist sees and although his/her opinion matters, yours does equally! If something really bugs you about your skin, you should be given the opportunity to talk about it openly, even if you are not sure whether there is a solution for this particular issue. For instance, you may be concerned about some dark pigmentation marks on your skin, and you might be thinking that nothing can be done about it. Wrong!

## 5. You are not being asked about your current skincare regime

Knowing your existing skincare regime does matter since what you apply to your skin will always affect your skin in a good or bad way. This will help identify gaps, mistakes or double-ups in the way you treat your skin. So, in order to help create a clear picture of your skincare regime, you should be asked plenty of questions starting with 'what', 'how' and 'when'. And, of course, the person that you are dealing with should also have a broad knowledge of all major skincare brands so they can relate to the products that you have been using.

## 6. You are not being offered a skin analysis

It is the role of your skincare professional to give you an accurate reading of your skin so you know which products are more likely to suit your skin. Is your skin normal, dry, oily, combination, dehydrated, sensitised? Although you might already know how your skin is, you should be able to get a confirmation of its current state (remember that your skin changes throughout the seasons, with your lifestyle, your stress levels, your state of health and with age).

## 7. You are feeling judged

Talking about your skin can be a very personal thing to do as it might involve sharing some private details about you and your life. It can also bring out some emotions, especially if your skin has been giving you trouble. This is why you need to connect with the right person for you, someone to whom you can express yourself freely and who understands where you are coming from. Someone who gets you!

## 8. You are feeling pressured to buy lots of products

You should be wary of anyone telling you to ditch all your current products (unless they can clearly explain a good rationale behind this recommendation, or if you really want to!) as the person you are dealing with might be more concerned about making a sale than actually helping you. Besides, it is usually best to introduce new products slowly, preferably no more than two or three at a time: this way, it is easier to pinpoint the source of the problem in case of an adverse reaction to the new products.

## 9. You are not given an explanation of how to use your new products

It is all very well to have the right skincare products, but you also need to know how and when to use them. Indeed, if used incorrectly, the best product can still be detrimental to your skin. For instance, if you are using too much of skin-refining ingredients (or too often, or for too long) such as fruit acids or retinol, you could potentially create skin damage and eventually accelerate skin ageing – the very thing that we want to alleviate. Ask for this information to be given to you in writing and in a step-by-step format, as all these new details could be a little overwhelming and quickly forgotten once you get home.

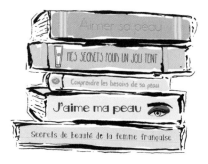

## The shelf life of your skincare products

Just like foods, skincare products are perishable items that eventually get denatured as they get exposed to light and oxygen, and through contamination by bacteria. Of course, all good skincare products should contain some ingredients that act as preservatives, but even the strongest of them cannot make a product last forever! All skincare products have a particular shelf life, which can be as long as two to three years from the time of manufacture or as short as one day (this is the case for some home-made artisan skincare products that contain food items such as fruits). The problem is that you rarely see expiry dates on skincare products and this makes it difficult to know how fresh the products you are buying really are.

**EXPERT TIPS**

Be aware of the fact that the shelf life of commercially produced, all-natural skincare products is always shorter (usually by half) than that of brands that use man-made and more stable preservative systems.

Always purchase your skincare from a reputable business that has a high product turnover and impeccable storage practices: this means rotating stock and displaying it in the darker and cooler area of the store (and NOT in the shop window!).

Some skincare brands give you an indication of the amount of time you can keep using their products once open: look for a little symbol that resembles an open jar with a specific number of months written on it. It should be displayed on the outer packaging.

Skincare products can be unsafe to use if contaminated: discontinue using a product that does not seem right to you, i.e. if it separates or has changed colour, or if it smells rancid or off.

Looking after your skincare products:

Keep in mind that you can shorten the shelf life of your products by handling them poorly. This is why you need to respect the following ground rules of skincare handling:

- Use a spatula (no fingers in jars!).
- Close lids properly after each use.
- Store products away from light.
- Store products in a cool place.

When I was little, Bonne Maman once taught me how not to handle skincare: 'Ne mets pas tes doigts dans mon pot de crème car tu vas la faire tourner,' she said, which means, 'Do not put your fingers in the jar, you are going to spoil my moisturiser.' Lesson learnt early.

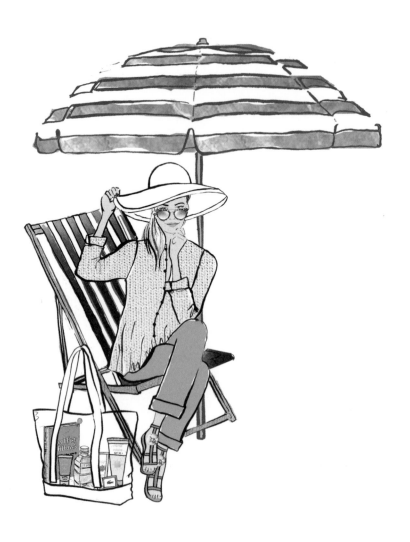

# CHAPTER 3

## CLEANSING, TONING, MOISTURISING AND USING SUN PROTECTION

As we know, skin requires a minimum of attention and care in order to thrive. In this chapter, let's have a look at the rationale and product specifics behind the ideal basic daily skincare routine that consists of cleansing, toning (optional), moisturising and using sun protection . . .

# Cleansing your skin

## The benefits of cleansing your skin

Cleansing your skin twice a day is a crucial step in your skincare regime that should be seen as being as important as brushing our teeth. Here are the reasons why: as our skin's rejuvenating activity peaks during the night, we need a morning cleanse to assist our largest organ with the removal of the excess toxins and sebum that have accumulated on it as we slept. And we need to cleanse again before bed time in order to completely remove the build-up of grime, excess oil, make-up and pollutants from our skin. By doing so, we can prevent (to a great extent) the occurrence of skin congestion and breakouts, and we can also boost the efficacy of our skincare by encouraging optimal absorption of the active ingredients present in products. In addition, a twice-daily cleanse encourages the blood and lymph flow around the facial area, which also contributes to our skin looking fresher.

## About cleansers

Cleansers come in different forms: oils, creams, milks, mousses, foaming washes, micellar waters etc. . . . But they have one thing in common: as just mentioned before, they need to be used twice a day every day!

## How to use your cleanser

Splash your face with lukewarm water first, or simply wet your hands before decanting your cleanser. Apply to your face, neck and décolletage. Gently massage for ten seconds or so, adding more water if you want to create more slip. If your skin is prone to congestion and breakouts, persist a little longer on these areas (usually the T-zone). Wipe clean with a wet cotton pad or fibrella (see expert tip below) and rinse well with water. If you are wearing heavy make-up, perform a 'double cleanse' by repeating this cleansing routine once more.

**EXPERT TIPS**

It does not matter how gentle your cleanser is, it should never be left on your skin! Unless you are using a micellar water (which does not need to be rinsed off), make sure to thoroughly wash your cleanser off with plenty of water so as to avoid drying out or clogging your skin.

Face washers are wonderful breeding grounds for bacteria in the tropical conditions of your bathroom: warm and humid! If you use one to cleanse your face, you'll need to change it at least daily, especially if you suffer from acne. Of course, this can be rather impractical. So, instead, use disposable items such as cotton pads or fibrellas to help remove traces of cleanser, grime and make-up from your skin.

Fibrellas are plain disposable facial wipes (not impregnated with any cleansing agent) that are used by many facialists to take products off their clients' skin during facial treatments. Use them wet, as you would use cotton pads, and discard after use. You can order fibrellas through a facialist.

## Common cleansing mistakes and misconceptions

*Thinking that cleansing your skin with water is enough*

Washing your skin with water alone does not constitute proper cleansing: you also need a cleanser to help break down all the grime, excess oil, make-up, toxins and pollutants that build up on the skin. Would we wash our dishes without dishwashing liquid? Of course not! Sorry, this is not a pretty analogy but I am sure you get my point: using a cleanser is necessary to maximise the cleansing property of water.

*Using harsh facial cleansers*

These days, I see a lot of women who use cleansers that are far too potent and far too stripping. The danger of using (or overusing) such cleansers lies in the fact that they can totally disturb the skin's natural quality and equilibrium: the skin starts to feel tight, it begins to look drier, and, over time, appears more lined. This usually leads to the need to overload the skin with heavier creams as a way to compensate, which can lead to unwanted skin congestion and breakouts, which, in turn, can lead to the temptation to use even harsher products as an attempt to clear the skin from those breakouts! This vicious circle could have been easily avoided by choosing a milder cleanser in the first place.

If you have inadvertently stripped your skin in this way, stop using the offending cleanser and swap it for one that has been specifically formulated for sensitive skin until your skin repairs itself and becomes more resilient. Whichever mild cleanser you go for, make sure that it is hypoallergenic, which means that it was formulated to minimise the risk of allergic reactions (I like the **La Roche-Posay Toleriane** range).

Once your skin has fully recovered, look for a milder cleanser than your original choice.

## Using soap on your face

Even if soap is rinsed off well and does not end up staying on the skin for very long, it still has the power to greatly affect its condition. In a sense, soap is too effective at cleansing the skin as it tends to remove too much of the natural oils which are essential to its good function and barrier integrity. Cleansing your face with soap can rapidly lead to skin dehydration, irritation and premature ageing. Not a good idea considering that our facial skin is constantly exposed to the elements and needs all the protection it can get!

## Believing that you need to use a facial cleansing device

As all my clients know, I have a profound aversion to all facial cleansing devices, including fancy electric brushes and manual cleansing pads and loofahs.

Firstly, as mentioned before, non-disposable items make a perfect party pad for bacteria (Moët & Chandon, anyone?) and should be disinfected on a daily basis. But who does that?

Secondly, the fact is that these facial devices can too easily become weapons of skin destruction. I have seen a lot of harm caused by using these cleverly marketed products: capillary damage (showing as red and blotchy skin) and skin dehydration (showing as fine lines that make your skin look older than it is) as well as skin irritation, all due to the over-stripping of the skin's protective oils and the removal of too many skin cells from the surface of the skin.

Lastly, you do not need any of these devices to achieve the perfect level of facial cleansing. Cleansing twice a day with a cleanser, your hands and some disposable cotton pads or fibrellas is the best and safest way to cleanse your face.

*Using facial cleansing wipes every day*

Cleansing wipes should only be used occasionally, if you really have to! They tend to be loaded with harsh cleansing agents, alcohol or fragrance (even the ones that are supposed to be for sensitive skin). So, having these sitting on your skin all day or all night is not the best idea! If you are time poor and want convenience, choose micellar water instead. More skin-friendly than cleansing wipes, micellar water is very popular in countries such as France where the water can be very hard and drying to the skin (this is why my grandmother always used to rinse her skin with rainwater). Called *lotion micellaire* in French, this type of ready-to-use cleanser works thanks to the gentle action of micelles (cleansing agents) and is designed to be applied onto a disposable cotton pad which you then wipe over your face until clean.

I personally like to use **Embryolisse Lotion Micellaire** as my all-in-one cleansing product (cleanser, eye and face make-up remover and toner) when I am in France. But as handy as wipes and micellar water can be, my view is that a rinse-off cleanser should always be your number-one and most frequent option, especially if your skin is prone to congestion and breaking out.

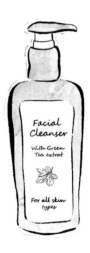

## Choosing the right cleanser

Cleansing with the right product is imperative: using a cleanser that is too harsh for your skin will lead to skin damage while using a product that is too rich will increase the likelihood of skin congestion and breakouts. You just need the right cleanser!

As a general rule, the thicker and richer a cleanser is (i.e. the higher its oil content), the more suitable it is for dehydrated, dry and/or mature skin. And the more foaming a cleanser is, the more suitable it is for an oilier skin type (although there is a new generation of foaming washes that are now specifically designed to be used on all skin types).

*A good way to know if your facial cleanser is the right one for you is to observe your skin after cleansing it: your skin should NOT feel tight, dry or uncomfortable as a result of cleansing it. Neither should it look devitalised or irritated.*

> **EXPERT TIP**
>
> Cleansing oils are currently very trendy. Yes, I do agree with the fact that they tend to smell lovely and that they leave the skin feeling extra soft but please, do not use them just because everyone else is! If you have oily skin, keep in mind that you will not benefit from using such cleansing oils since they can encourage clogging and breakouts. In this case, you are better off using a light cleansing milk or a non-stripping cleansing gel. Leave cleansing oils for those with drier skin types or wait until you are older (when your skin will have become less oily).

# Late teens and twenties cleanser recommendations

At this age, your skin is likely to be prone to breakouts and congestion (it may look 'bumpy' with pimples, blackheads and whiteheads) due to your hormones going a little crazy! If this is the case, resist the urge to use harsh and stripping cleansers as these will NOT improve your complexion. What will benefit your skin the most is regularity, which means cleansing your face every morning and every night.

## Skin Juice Eden Smoothing Cleansing Cream (Origin: Australia)

The main reason why I like this light and creamy cleanser is that it helps purify the skin without disturbing its natural balance: it discourages skin congestion (thanks to the presence of mildly exfoliating fruit and milk acids) while helping to maintain your skin moisture levels so you do not end up looking like a dried-out prune (or *pruneau* in French). This product best suits normal to oily skin types.

## Image Skincare Ormedic Balancing Facial Cleanser (Origin: USA)

This is an excellent rebalancing foaming wash (and yet non-stripping) that was formulated with all skin types in mind. I consider it to be one of my greatest finds as it has helped countless clients of mine from various age groups (including many acne sufferers) achieve their goal of having clear, smooth and healthy-looking skin.

# Thirties cleanser recommendations

If you are in your thirties, you are most likely to be time poor (and this is probably an understatement!). You may be a new mum and/or you might be establishing yourself professionally. You could even be studying while working. In any case, you know all too well that time is a rare commodity and that facial cleansing will not feature on your extensive to-do list unless it can be done quickly and easily. The following cleansers are *très pratiques* (French for very convenient!) and can be used under the shower to save even more time.

## Sircuit Skin Cosmeceuticals Supermild Sensitive Skin Cleansing Crème (Origin: USA)

This is a gentle yet effective wash that is suitable for all skin types. It initially looks like a cream but transforms into a light foaming cleanser once you mix it with water (if it does not foam, you have not used enough water). Don't be fooled by its name or its smooth texture: 'Supermild' is a gentle and yet tough operator that quickly dissolves grime and make-up without much effort on your part. It is also a very economical product as a little goes a very long way.

## Institut Esthederm Osmoclean Pure Cleansing Foam (Origin: France)

This is a ready-to-use cleanser for combination and oily skin. It allows for a quick and thorough facial cleanse without stripping the skin. You just need to apply a couple of pumps' worth of this foam onto your wet skin, massage lightly for ten seconds max, splash your face with water and *voilà!* It is done!

# Forties cleanser recommendations

As your skin is maturing, it might be time to swap your existing cleanser for a more hydrating one and to choose a product designed for normal to dry or dehydrated skin. Note to yourself: a well-hydrated skin will always look younger!

### Institut Esthederm Osmoclean Hydra-Replenishing Cleansing Milk (Origin: France)

The name says it all! This cleanser gives the skin a real moisture boost while cleansing it. This is a good product to introduce if you swear by facial cleansing gels and are reluctant to move on to a cleansing milk, as it is still light and non-greasy. This means that it will not make you feel like you need another cleanser to wash off your cleanser! Just a little water will suffice to give you that nice clean feel.

### Uskincare Nourish Milk Cleanser (Origin: Australia)

This is one of my Aussie favourites with a lovely citrusy scent! An unpretentious and yet very reliable cleansing milk that is full of quality ingredients, all contributing to its gentle and yet thorough cleansing action. The camellia oil present in this cleanser deserves a high distinction for its excellent protective, hydrating and softening action on the skin. All in all, Nourish Milk Cleanser adds a real pleasurable dimension to facial cleansing.

# Fifties and beyond cleanser recommendations

This is the time in your life when you are seeing your body and your skin change, and not necessarily the way you would want them to! *Oh mon Dieu* (OMG): your waistline is wanting to expand at an exponential rate and your skin is now showing more wrinkles! Extra nurturing is what you and your skin needs right now.

## Skin Juice Drench Dermal Repair Cleansing Oil (Origin: Australia)

Cleansing oils can bring instant comfort to the skin but you must choose them carefully as oils ain't oils! Why would you want to use a cleansing oil that has mineral oil (petroleum derived) as its main ingredient when your skin could benefit from natural, antioxidant rich, plant-based oils? Drench Dermal Repair Cleansing Oil is one of the latter. It is also a refined water-soluble formulation (based on healing macadamia and carrot-seed oils) that does not leave your skin feeling greasy, just nicely hydrated and conditioned. Not to mention its exquisite smell! This product is best suited for combination, dry and dehydrated skin types.

## Sothys Beauty Garden Make-Up Removing Fluid (Origin: France)

If cleansing with oil is not your thing, you might prefer Beauty Garden Make-Up Removing Fluid, which is part of Sothys' certified organic collection, and which is suitable for all skin types. This light cleansing milk contains a plant-based moisturising complex designed to strengthen the skin's barrier function and increase hydration. Clinical tests performed by the University of Limoges, located south-west of Paris, confirm the validity of this claim.

# Toning your skin

## The benefits of toning your skin

Although toners are marketed as being essential for restoring the skin's normal pH after cleansing, your skin will eventually do this by itself. This means that you do not really have to tone unless you have sensitive, irritated and/or dry skin.

However, if you are like me, you might like to use a toner anyway, to complement your facial cleansing, regardless of your skin type or condition.

## About toners

Toners come in different categories based on their effects on the skin: hydrating, soothing or astringent (which means tightening to the skin).

- A hydrating toner can help rehydrate dehydrated skin.
- A soothing toner can bring relief to sensitive or sensitised skin.
- An astringent toner can help purify oily skin.

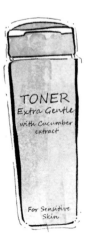

## How to use your toner

Put a little toner onto a disposable cotton pad (no need to saturate, use just enough toner so the cotton pad feels slightly wet). Wipe the cotton pad over your entire face, neck and décolletage, or on a localised area only (depending on the type of toner you are using, and your skin type and condition).

### EXPERT TIPS

If you are time poor and want to save on your toning time, you might prefer to spritz your hydrating or soothing toner. To do this, decant some of your favourite product into an empty spray bottle, which you should find at most pharmacies or department stores (they are usually sold for travel).

You can also carry this spray bottle of toner with you and refresh your skin at any time over the course of the day. This is particularly recommended if you wear mineral make-up, as regular misting of your skin will help maintain a more dewy finish.

## Common toning mistakes and misconceptions

### *Mistaking the property of your toner*

I regularly meet women who use a particular mass-marketed witch-hazel toner, thinking that it will soothe their dry or sensitive skin. It is true that witch hazel is a plant that has anti-inflammatory and calming properties (on top of its mild astringent qualities). However, most of the witch hazel–based toners available on the market are strong astringent products that are formulated with other ingredients such as alcohol or salicylic acid, and this makes them far too harsh and drying for most skin types.

If you are after a very gentle and soothing witch hazel–based toner for all skin types, try **Embryolisse Eau de Beauté Rosamélis**. For a more powerful astringent (but still very skin friendly!), try alcohol-free **Gernetic Fibro**, which is for all skin types except sensitised skin.

### *Using heavily fragranced toners*

Heavily fragranced toners can irritate the skin. Furthermore, when combined with sun exposure, they can cause your skin to become sensitised and to develop dark pigmentation marks (called hyperpigmentation). These risks not only apply to synthetic fragrances but they are also associated with some natural essential oils (beware of citrusy oils including bergamot). For this reason, it is best to choose a fragrance-free or subtly fragranced toner. Natural floral waters are always a good option as they are diluted products (they contain essential oils but in a much lesser concentration). You may also want to opt for mineral water sprays, such are those by **La Roche-Posay** or **Evian** in summer months.

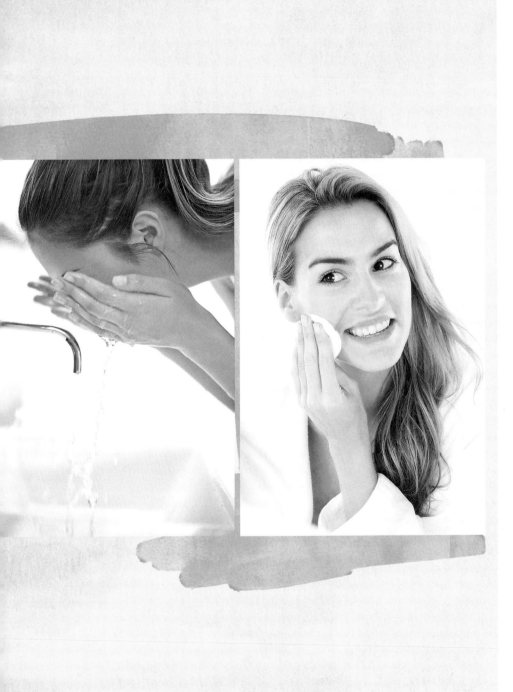

# Late teens and twenties toner recommendations

It is very easy to get caught up in the hype and fall for brands that promise you the world. This is particularly the case for products that are supposed to clear your blemishes overnight and forever. Do not believe such claims! These harsh products will not help your skin but will most certainly completely dry it out and cause some irritation. If this has happened to you, throw these products away and use a skin-friendly toner as a way to help heal, soothe and rehydrate your skin. Once this is achieved, you can then move on to an alcohol-free astringent toner.

## Institut Esthederm Osmoclean Alcohol Free Calming Lotion (Origin: France)

This is a good emergency toner for any skin that has been stripped and sensitised. Fragrance-free and packed with moisturising ingredients, it will help soothe, repair and rehydrate your skin so it can resume its natural function of protection. *Traitons notre peau avec douceur!* (Meaning, let's treat our skin gently!)

## Skin Juice Multi Juice Balancing Tonic (Origin: Australia)

It is only once your skin's natural barrier function has been fortified that you can start using a gentle astringent toner such as Multi Juice Balancing Tonic. This product contains pink grapefruit, lime and lemon myrtle extracts which all help to purify the skin and keep breakouts under control. And unlike some other toners that are meant to help clear blemish-prone skin, this toner will not make your skin look and feel like sandpaper since its main ingredient is aloe vera (and it contains no alcohol).

# Thirties toner recommendations

I know how busy you are but I sincerely hope that you are managing to keep up with your skincare rituals. That: 1. you are cleansing your skin twice a day; and 2. you are using a proper rinse-off cleanser for it. But just in case you cannot resist the temptation of using cleansing wipes (you know how I feel about them!), here is a chance to do your skin a good turn: use a toner to wash away all the unwanted detergent residues that should not be left on your face. Your toner can be the next best thing to water!

## Sukin Hydrating Mist Toner (Origin: Australia)

Spritz, spritz, spritz! And let the gentle effects of rosewater and German chamomile combine to cleanse, soothe and refresh your skin. This is a good quality and inexpensive facial mist that also helps restore moisture. It can be used at any time of the day, anywhere and on any skin type.

## Gernetic Fibro (Origin: France)

As seen previously, Fibro is a mildly astringent toner that is suitable for all skin types except sensitised skin. It also makes a great eye and lip make-up remover (it removes most waterproof make-up products). You could even use this toner to make your own cleansing wipe: a cotton pad with some Fibro on it: *voilà*! A lovely wipe with a refreshing blend of chamomile, ginseng, lime, cucumber and witch-hazel extracts. Will you ditch your other manufactured facial wipes? *Oui? S'il vous plaît!*

# Forties toner recommendations

In addition to using a moisturiser, using a toner can be a very effective way to help boost your skin's hydration level (in my 20-plus years spent treating skin, I have never seen a single face that was *too* hydrated!). There are a lot of great hydrating toners on the market, but I find that the two below-mentioned products are particularly worth the expense as they do work absolute wonders on the skin. These are real aid workers for anybody who wants more radiant looking skin and are my hand-picked selection if you are in your forties (or beyond: I am still using them!).

## Institut Esthederm Cellular Water Spray (Origin: France)

This is not just a water spray! Fundamental to the entire Esthederm range, its chemical composition mimics the water that is naturally found in our skin. This similarity results in a healthier-looking and energised complexion. This product is to be used on clean skin.

## Sircuit Skin Cosmeceuticals Molecular Mist (Origin: USA)

If you are after long-lasting hydration, you cannot go past Molecular Mist. It literally feels and acts like a liquid moisturiser on your skin. Added bonuses: its packaging is totally travel resistant which means that it will not leak in your handbag. And, as it is available in a 60ml non-aerosol spray, you can take it flying with you. In fact, it is always with me on those long-haul flights to France. A real skin rescue solution!

# Fifties and beyond toner recommendations

In our fifties and beyond, our blood capillaries start losing their elasticity, which can make our skin more prone to flushing. Some toners can alleviate some of the resulting redness and heat by helping soothe and cool the skin. Not to mention the added hydration that they provide to our skin. Yes please!

## Uskincare Damask Rose Hydrosol (Origin: Australia)

Bulgarian rose petals and gotu kola extracts make this product a particularly soothing toner. Its rich (and yet ephemeral) rose aroma is reminiscent of those exquisitely manicured European gardens. A few mists and there you are, walking the grounds around the Chateau de Versailles!

## Embryolisse Eau de Beauté Rosamélis (Origin: France)

Recommended for all skin types including sensitive, this hydrating toner is infused with a soothing blend of rose, cornflower and orange flowers, all adding to the softness of this formulation and to its beautiful natural scent. It feels like a caress on your skin. Lovely!

# Using eye care products

## The benefits of using eye care products

The skin of the eye area is very fine and delicate. It is also under enormous stress, not only from our constant facial movements but also from being exposed to environmental pollution and climate aggressors such as air dryness and UV radiation. All of this makes our eye contour more prone to premature ageing, hence the need for extra care and protection!

## About eye care products

Eye care products include eye make-up removers (waterproof and non-waterproof) and a variety of eye treatment products ranging form eye gels to oils. Please note that I have intentionally left out eye contour oils simply because I do not believe in using pure oils as an eye treatment, even when they have specifically been formulated for this area. I find oils to be too heavy for the fine and delicate skin of the eye contour: they tend to encourage the appearance of milia and often make eye puffiness worse.

## How to use your eye care products

### Eye make-up remover

Squeeze a little eye make-up remover onto a cotton pad. Place onto one eye and gently press onto the skin for a few seconds (this will help dissolve your eye make-up). Wipe over the eye contour, turn your cotton pad over and wipe again to complete your eye make-up removal. Repeat the same process on your other eye, using a fresh cotton pad.

**EXPERT TIP**

If your eye make-up remover is dual-phased (i.e. containing oil and water), make sure to shake the bottle well before each use so you don't have the oil part floating on top. You need to use the entire formulation and not only the oil component.

*Eye gel or eye cream*

After you have cleansed and toned your skin, place a small amount of your eye gel or cream onto your ring fingers and gently dab onto the eye contour: start under the eye, over the orbital bone (the eye socket) from the inner to the outer corner of the eye, and back again. Move your fingers under your eyebrow, and gently glide them over the brow bone from the inner to the outer corner.

## EXPERT TIPS

Gentle patting of the eye contour helps with the absorption of your eye gel or cream. It also stimulates the microcirculation around the eyes, which can have a noticeable de-puffing effect.

To add to the decongesting effect of an eye gel or cream, cool it down before use (put it in your refrigerator). The cold temperature will encourage your capillaries to contract and as a result will help shift some of the excess fluid that causes eye puffiness.

Whatever you use on your eyes, be gentle!

## Common eye care mistakes and misconceptions

*Using non-specific eye products around the eye area*

Products not intended for use over the eye contour might have ingredients that could potentially irritate your eyes and cause the appearance of milia (round whitish bumps that can sometimes be felt under the skin) or even styes (ouch! This happened to me once!). So it is best to avoid using any face product that is not clearly marketed as being suitable for the eye contour.

*Using too much of your eye gel or eye cream*

Half a pea-sized amount of product is more than enough for both eyes. Using more is a waste and can lead to puffiness (especially with eye creams) as you overload the delicate skin of the eye contour. This may also result in the formation of milia.

*Applying your eye gel or eye cream too close to the eyes*

As our skin warms up over the course of the day, skincare products that we have applied tend to become more fluid. This means that an eye gel or eye cream initially applied too close to the eyes is likely to seep into them. This is sometimes the reason why people believe that they cannot tolerate eye products. But these are not meant to go in the eyes, just over the eye contour. (If you still feel like your eyes are too sensitive to use any eye product at all, try this last option: **Institut Esthederm Sensi System Calming Eye Contour Cream.** This is the most soothing and highly tolerated eye cream I know of.)

All skincare products used around the eye area should be of the utmost quality and freshness so as to eliminate any potential risk of allergic reaction or infection, which could have dangerous consequences for the eye itself.

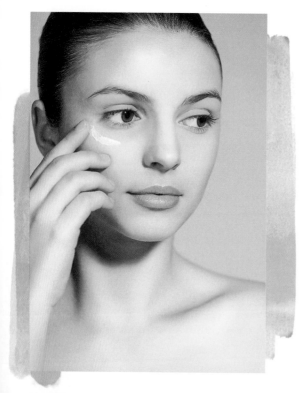

## Choosing the right eye care products

### *Eye make-up remover*

These days, most facial cleansers can be used around the eye area. However, it is best to use a specific eye make-up remover to properly remove eye make-up.

### *Eye gel or eye cream*

Traditionally, eye gels assist with puffiness and dark circles while eye creams usually target the visual signs of ageing (fine lines and wrinkles). But things are changing: the last few years have seen the emergence of a new generation of eye gels and creams that address all concerns at once. These can be handy if you do not want to use two different eye treatment products.

Which eye make-up remover should you choose?

Do no select your eye-make up remover according to your age but rather based on the type of eye make-up that you wear.

For non-waterproof make-up: use a gentle eye make-up remover such as *The Body Shop Camomile Gentle Eye Make-up Remover.*

For waterproof eye make-up: dual-phase removers work best. The classic *Clarins Instant Eye Make-up Remover* will remove the most stubborn eye make-up effortlessly. However, if your eyes are very susceptible to irritation, you might want to choose an unfragranced product such as *Institut Esthederm Osmoclean High Tolerance Make-up Remover - Waterproof Eyes and Lips,* which is also very effective.

# Late teens and twenties eye care recommendations

In your late teens and twenties, using an eye gel or eye cream every day is not truly necessary unless you are already wearing eye make-up regularly. In this case, a little tender loving care is advisable to help protect and hydrate your eye contour. Gel or cream? Your pick!

## Uskincare Revital Eyes Eyelift Gel (Origin: Australia)

This is a light, aloe vera–based gel that feels very cooling on the eye contour. It contains eyebright (to fight puffiness and dark circles), camellia oil (to lightly protect and nourish) and rosehip oil (to minimise the ageing action of those nasty free radicals). Revital Eyes Eyelift Gel is a wonderful all-rounder.

## Clarins Eye Contour Balm (Origin: France)

For an eye treatment with a little more 'body' choose a product that contains shea butter, such as this one. Eye Contour Balm also works well at soothing overworked eyes. Those long hours spent on the computer studying . . . or Facebooking . . . this balm works equally well in both cases!

# Thirties eye care recommendations

In your thirties, your eyes are starting to show more signs of fatigue and your hectic lifestyle is not helping! This is why you need to invest in slightly more active eye treatment products that can brighten your eye contour, target its first signs of ageing and strongly protect it against excessive free radical damage.

## Bliss Triple Oxygen Instant Energizing Eye Gel (Origin: Switzerland)

This is an eye gel with character and substance! It decongests and brightens the eye contour thanks to its caffeine and vitamin C content. I like the fact that it leaves a slight emollient film on the skin (this could eliminate the need to use a separate eye cream if you prefer to use a single product). Also worth a mention is the presence of soft-focus powders to reflect light and instantly blur fine lines and wrinkles.

## Antipodes Kiwi Seed Oil Eye Cream (Origin: New Zealand)

I first discovered the Antipodes range at a beauty trade fair in Paris years ago when it was still an unknown brand and I am very pleased to see how well established this company now is. I particularly like their Kiwi Seed Oil Eye Cream: a light moisturiser for the eye contour with an ingredient mix scientifically tested and shown to stimulate the production of collagen in the skin.

# Forties eye care recommendations

Now is the time to bring out the big guns! Cosmeceutical-strength eye care is what your eye contour needs to not only reduce dark circles and puffiness (by encouraging the local microcirculation) but also to restore youth. There are many good choices out there but these two eye serums are absolutely worth mentioning. If you want to select your own options, look for products with similar active ingredients that may give you comparable results.

## Epicure Cosmeceuticals Skin Firming Eye Serum (Origin: Australia)

I have been getting impressive results with Skin Firming Eye Serum, which I have been using as my eye care product for the last three months. Containing a high-tech blend of decongesting and firming active ingredients (green-coffee extract, Eyeseryl, Bioskinup and Haloxyl), this eye serum has helped to substantially diminish the signs of fatigue that have developed around these tired eyes.

## Sircuit Skin Cosmeceuticals White Out Daily Under Eye Care (Origin: USA)

This is a unique eye product that specifically targets under-eye puffiness and dark circles with the help of active ingredients such as Eyeliss, Haloxyl and magnolia extract. I like the addition of a mild fruit-acid blend to help smooth and renew the skin. Another plus: White Out Daily Under Eye Care contains zinc oxide to add to its calming and protective dimension, as well as some light-dispersing particles to even out the colour of the skin.

# Fifties and beyond eye care recommendations

In your fifties and beyond your eye contour can greatly benefit from the synergetic actions of time-tested natural elements and cosmetic science. In these two examples, marine elements (criste marine plant extracts and sea water concentrate) and liquid crystals are utilised to deeply nourish, smooth and protect the skin around the eye.

## Phytomer Expertise Age Contour Intense Youth Eye Cream (Origin: France)

This protective eye cream is packed with restorative ingredients: marine trace elements, minerals, shea butter, hyaluronic acid and antioxidants. Note that it is a light-textured product. If you prefer a more unctuous cream, choose . . .

## Epicure Cosmeceuticals Anti-Ageing Eye Serum: Liquid Crystal (Origin: Australia)

This eye serum should really be called an eye cream: it has an incredibly rich and smooth texture that helps create a protective and repairing shield over the eye contour. Liquid crystals contribute to its moisturising effects, and they also give this eye care product its beautiful changing colour (yes, they are true liquid crystals!). I personally prefer to use this product at night as I find that it looks a little too shimmery for day use.

# Moisturising your skin

## The benefits of using a moisturiser

EXCELLENT NEWS: no matter what skin type you have, it will always look younger when it is hydrated. For this reason, moisturising can make us look much more youthful (super!).

Using a moisturiser can also help reinforce the barrier function of our skin by maintaining the right balance of oil and moisture at epidermis level. And it is an easy way to 'feed' our skin with some protective or repairing ingredients such as antioxidants or peptides.

## About moisturisers

There are two main types of moisturising agents in face creams: emollients and humectants.

### Emollients

Emollients are fatty ingredients that create a protective 'blanket' over the epidermis: instead of being evaporated from the skin, water remains trapped under this emollient film where it is then able to rehydrate the skin's outer layer. Emollients also make the skin more supple. Common skincare ingredients with emollient properties are squalene, mineral oil, shea butter, almond oil, jojoba oil and coconut oil.

### Humectants

Humectants work by bonding with water molecules from the air and the skincare that we apply on our skin, and this leads to an increase in the water content of our epidermis. Common skincare ingredients with humectant properties are glycerin, sodium PCA, propylene glycol, natural moisturising factor (NMF) and, one of my very favourite moisture-binding and skin-plumping skincare ingredients: hyaluronic acid (a definite must have!).

## How to use your moisturiser

Place a little moisturiser onto your fingertips – usually a pea-sized amount for the face and neck, and a little more for the décolletage. Note that this amount may vary depending on the product used and the condition of your skin. Press your fingertips onto your cheeks, forehead, chin, neck and décolletage to deposit the moisturiser evenly around your skin. Spread the moisturiser over the skin until all areas are covered.

> **EXPERT TIP**
>
> If your moisturiser is a very rich emollient cream that is harder to spread, warm it up first before applying it to your face: place a small amount of cream onto your fingertips and rub together before pressing it onto all areas of skin that you want to treat.

## Common moisturising mistakes and misconceptions

### *Confusing exfoliating and renewing creams with moisturisers*

A cream that contains a high level of fruit acids should be regarded as an exfoliant and a vitamin A–based cream should be regarded as a skin renewing product, full stop. A moisturiser should be moisturising (what a scoop!) so if you are using a cream that makes your skin feel tight and dry, check its ingredients as it is most likely to contain such corrective agents. To identify a moisturiser, look for words such as 'moisturising', 'hydrating' or 'nourishing' on the packaging.

### *Using the same amount of moisturiser all over*

Most of us do not have the same skin type all over. Usually, the T-zone tends to be a little oilier than the rest of your face, and may require less moisturising than your cheeks, for instance. This is why you should judge and control the amount of cream that you apply to different areas of your skin. To do this, moisturise the driest areas first and finish where your skin is oilier.

### *Forgetting your neck and décolletage*

As your neck and décolletage are usually as exposed to the elements as your face, they need an equal level of care. This is why they should also be included into your daily skincare routine.

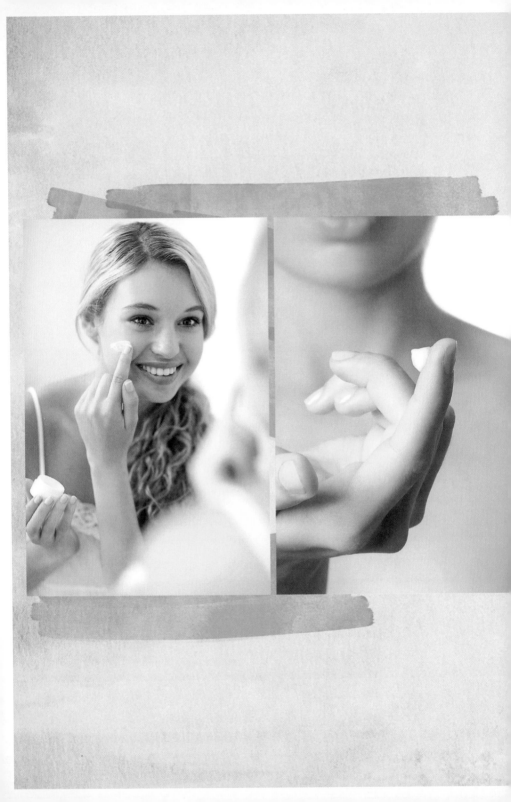

## Choosing the right moisturiser

Emollient-based creams are richer and thicker in texture than humectant-based moisturisers. As a rule, creams that are designed for an oilier skin type will always have more humectants than emollients. On the contrary, moisturisers for dry skins will be richer in emollients.

These days, most face creams are designed for both day and night use except for the ones that have strong corrective actives (such as fruit acids or retinol), which should preferably be used at night.

It can be difficult to choose the right moisturiser from the myriad of products available out there. Remember, the lighter the texture of a moisturiser, the more suited it is for an oilier skin type.

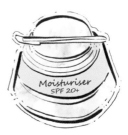

# Late teens and twenties moisturiser recommendations

By now you should have got into the habit of moisturising your skin every day. If you have not yet, come on, now is the time! Did you know that the sheer fact of using a moisturiser can prevent your skin from getting breakouts by keeping it more balanced and supple?

## Sukin Facial Moisturiser (Origin: Australia)

This moisturiser suits all skin types. It is packed with skin healing and protecting ingredients such as aloe, rosehip, jojoba seed oil and vitamin E. This light moisturiser also has a subtle scent that is absolutely divine: citrusy sweet with notes of vanilla, tangerine and mandarin. Added bonus: its low price.

## Skin Juice Citrus Oil Control Face Cream (Origin: Australia)

This is a non-clogging, lightweight moisturiser for oily and combination skin types that have a tendency to breakouts. Citrus Oil Control Face Cream contains ingredients that have skin rebalancing and soothing properties (Reguseb complex, manuka and arctic cranberry), which all contribute to making the skin look clearer and brighter.

# Thirties moisturiser recommendations

You may have started to notice your first lines and wrinkles appearing on your face. Do not panic! It is time to choose a moisturiser with extra water-binding properties. Remember: no matter what skin type you have, it will always look younger when it is hydrated. Does this sound too simple to be true? Well, it is true! Try it for yourself and you will see. Your skin can never have too much moisture. *Vive l'hydratation!*

## Indeed Laboratories Hydraluron Moisture Jelly (Origin: Canada)

This hyaluronic acid–based gel is a true humectant product with fantastic hydrating properties. Hydraluron Moisture Jelly is suitable for all skin types (although people with dry skin would need to apply another cream on top). It is great for men too as it does not make your skin look shiny.

## Institut Esthederm Hydra System Aqua Diffusion Care Cream (Origin: France)

This moisturiser can be used on all skin types. It has a well-rounded texture that makes it both light and creamy. Hydra System Aqua Diffusion Care Cream leaves the skin looking super plump and moisturised without being too heavy, which makes it a good base for a long-lasting make-up finish.

# Forties moisturiser recommendations

Your forties is the right time to introduce a moisturiser with a little more body since your skin is now maturing and in need of more substantial products. Choosing a cream with a higher emollient content (remember those lovely fats and oils!) will ensure that your skin gets the extra nourishment and protection that it now needs. A friendly reminder: make sure to change cleansers too. If you have not already, please refer to the previous section on cleansers. *Très important!*

## Auriège Paris Chrono-V Revitalizing Global Care (Origin: France)
This is a good moisturiser for ageing skin that needs more protection without too much nourishment as it has the right balance of humectants and emollients. Chrono-V Revitalizing Global Care is enriched with vitamins, which add to this cream's replenishing and protective effects. It has a lovely creamy texture and a pleasant scent that is reminiscent of a classic French *crème pour le visage* (face cream).

## Embryolisse Lait-Crème Concentré (Origin: France)
While I would not recommend this cream to someone with combination or oily skin, it works well on dry or very dehydrated skin. If you are someone who likes simplicity and who is not into using a lot of skincare products, this would be the ideal product for you since you can also use this moisturiser as a primer, a facial mask, and even as an emergency make-up remover! A very handy product that is much loved by make-up artists around the world.

# Fifties and beyond moisturiser recommendations

This is a time where your skin is likely to feel and look much drier than before due to a drop in your hormone levels and a decrease in the activity of your sebaceous glands (which are now producing less oil). This affects your skin's ability to hold on to moisture. This is why you may need to change moisturiser and choose a much richer one. However, if you are still prone to getting the odd blemish (like me!), there is no need for you to use a heavier cream every day. In this case, you would only need to do this when you feel like your skin needs a little bit more conditioning, and would alternate with a lighter cream.

## Epicure Cosmeceuticals Intensive Care Hydrator (Origin: Australia)

This cream suits dry, dehydrated, ageing and mature skin particularly well. It is enriched with shea butter, which contributes to its pleasant texture and its good skin-soothing properties. Rich in antioxidants, Intensive Care Hydrator is also a deliciously scented product (peach!).

## Gernetic Cytobi (Origin: France)

Cytobi is the most nourishing and healing cream I know of (Gernetic skincare was initially created to be used in the burns unit of a Paris hospital by French biologist Albert Laporte). It has a very rich texture and only a very small amount is needed (and should be used) to feed the driest of skin! This is a truly amazing moisturiser for dry or mature skin.

# Using sun protection

## The benefits of sun protection

Sunlight is essential to our general health: emotionally, a little sunshine has the ability to make us feel better and lift our spirits, and on a physical level, we need some sun on our skin to synthesise vitamin D so we can remain generally healthy. But all is not rosy under the sun (no pun intended!). UV radiation from the sun (and tanning beds) can cause skin cancers and photo-ageing. Unfortunately, this UV-related skin damage can occur without giving us any warning: unlike UVB rays, UVA rays rarely make our skin burn. Nevertheless, UVA radiation can lead to serious DNA damage and severe wrinkling of the skin since its rays penetrate deeper into the skin than UVBs. (Did you know that tanning beds mainly emit UVA radiation? Grrrr, I loathe them!)

In Australia, there is a growing awareness of the link between UV exposure and skin cancer, thanks to the very effective Cancer Council's SunSmart campaign that encourages people to 'Slip, Slop, Slap, Seek and Slide'. This slogan stands for: 'Slip on protective clothing, Slop on SPF 30 or higher sunscreen, Slap on a hat, Seek shade and Slide on some sunnies' (www.sunsmart.com.au/uv-sun-protection/uv). Unfortunately, there are still too many people who fail to recognise that UV radiation can also precipitate skin ageing. And this is a shame, considering that photo-ageing can be so easily avoided.

*If skin cancer does not scare you, think 'skin ageing' and let vanity lead you to a tube of sunscreen!*

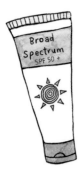

In 2014, I had the great pleasure of personally meeting Australian Professor Adele Green at the Anti-Ageing Skin Care Conference at the Royal College of Physicians in London where she had been invited to present the results of her long world-renowned research on the anti-ageing effect of sunscreen on the skin. Adele explained her work: a randomised, controlled trial (regarded as the gold standard for clinical research) which took place in Nambour, a small town located in very sunny Queensland. It involved a healthy local population of 903 adults (male and female) under the age of fifty-five. One group was instructed to use a supplied broad-spectrum 15+ sunscreen daily while the other group was told to use sunscreen in a discretionary manner, as they normally would (i.e. mostly sporadically or not at all).

After four and a half years, results showed that the research participants belonging to the daily sunscreen group displayed 24 per cent less skin ageing compared with those in the discretionary sunscreen group. (M.C.B. Hughes, G.M. Williams, P. Baker & A.C. Green, 'Sunscreen and Prevention of Skin Aging: A Randomized Trial', *Annals of Internal Medicine*, 2013; 158:781–790)

## PHOTO-AGEING WARNINGS

While all skin types are susceptible to photo-ageing, people with fairer skin (like myself) – naturally pale skin that can easily get sunburnt and can hardly tan – are more prone to showing even stronger signs of photo-ageing if they are not sun smart.

Photo-ageing may not show up instantly. Damage can appear much later in life. So do not think that you have been spared! Repeated and prolonged exposure to UV radiation (from the sun OR TANNING BEDS) will eventually manifest, as described below. So, it is time to get real and to implement the very smart Australian Cancer Council's SunSmart guidelines: 'Slip, Slop, Slap, Seek and Slide'.

Do not forget to protect your children too.

## The visible signs of photo-ageing

Photo-ageing negatively affects our skin at every level and its visible signs are always much more severe and obvious than those of chronological ageing. In other words, sun damaged skin will always look older than skin of the same age that has not been exposed to as much UV radiation.

*On photo-aged skin:*

- lines and wrinkles are more pronounced
- skin sagging is more obvious
- skin is thicker and more 'leathery' looking
- dilated blood capillaries are likely to be more prominent
- uneven pigmentation is more frequent
- solar keratoses (pre-cancerous lesions that appear as little dry-looking crusts on the surface of the skin) may appear
- skin cancers are much more likely to develop.

Take the photo-ageing test

The best way to judge the visible difference between natural ageing and photo-ageing is to observe and compare your facial skin with the skin on areas that have been less exposed to the sun (such as your buttocks or your tummy).

Look at the difference: can you see some signs of photo-ageing on your face?

An example of intensely photo-aged skin is that of Brigitte Bardot, now in her eighties, who, in her younger days, spent a lot of time sunbaking on the French Riviera. The ageing effect of prolonged and cumulative sun exposure on Bardot's face becomes even more evident when you compare her with someone like Anouk Aimée, another French actress of a similar age. (Having said that, I totally admire Brigitte Bardot's choice to shun plastic surgery and her total dedication to worldwide animal rights. Bravo Brigitte!)

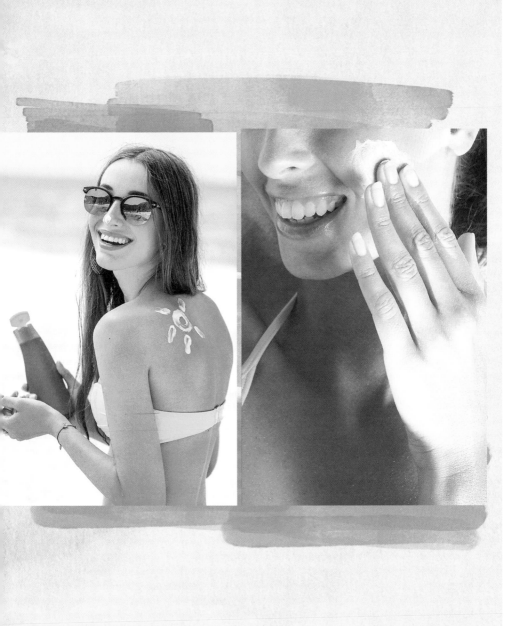

## About sunscreen

Sunscreens are skincare products that are specifically designed to protect the skin against the damaging effects of UV radiation. For this reason, they are classified as therapeutic products and not as cosmetics.

Although moisturisers with SPF are not considered as 'true' sunscreens (since their primary function is to moisturise the skin), these cosmetic products can also be a good option to help prevent some of the skin damage caused by UV radiation.

Sunscreen actives work in two ways: either by reflecting light – as in the case of physical sunscreen ingredients such as zinc oxide and titanium dioxide – or by absorbing and neutralising UV rays – as in the case of chemical sunscreen ingredients such as octyl methoxycinnamate, oxybenzone, avobenzone and many others.

> Whichever active ingredients your sun protection product contains, always remember that a water-resistant, broad spectrum sunscreen (UVA and UVB protection) with a high SPF will give you the best sun protection. Look out for these details on the packaging of sunscreens.

Did you know that . . .

SPF stands for Sun Protection Factor. It indicates a sunscreen's level of protection against UVB radiation.

'Broad spectrum' refers to the scope of a sunscreen's UV protection and means that it filters both UVA and UVB radiation.

## When and how to use your sunscreen

The World Health Organization (WHO) stipulates that we should all use sunscreen on days when the UV index for the area we live in reaches 3 or above: this is the level where UV radiation is considered to be damaging (ageing!) to the skin and conducive to skin cancer. An extreme level of solar radiation is considered to be reached when the UV index gets up to 11 and beyond.

For maximum sun protection, apply your sunscreen directly on clean skin (like a face moisturiser but in a much more liberal fashion), at least 20 minutes before going out in the sun so it has time to settle and activate on your skin. If spending the day in the sun, reapply every two hours (or more if you sweat profusely or if you have been in water).

The World Health Organization website (www.who.int/uv/) publishes a list of UV index reporting sites throughout the world.

If you live in Australia, where you have to be so careful about sun exposure, download the free SunSmart mobile app (available for Android and iPhone). An initiative of SunSmart Victoria, this app keeps you informed about the current UV index wherever you are and the hours during which you should avoid sun exposure. It also allows you to create a personalised profile and find out exactly how much sunscreen you need to apply. It even has a tracker so you know how much daily sun exposure you require to keep your vitamin D levels in a healthy range. Oh, and you can even get alerts sent to your phone. Just brilliant!

Do not think that you are safe if the weather is overcast. I remember a recent summer day in Australia: it was very hot, but the sun was hiding behind a barrage of thick clouds. I was trying to guess the UV index, which I thought could be around 4. To be sure, I checked on my phone (using my newly discovered SunSmart app) and was shocked to see CURRENT UV: 10! Thankfully, I was wearing sunscreen.

Note that using a sunscreen does not make you vitamin D deficient and that you do not usually need a lot of time in the sun to build the required levels of vitamin D. But if you are worried about a deficiency in vitamin D, consult your doctor and ask to have your levels checked.

## Common sun protection mistakes and misconceptions

### *Not using enough sunscreen*

As I mentioned previously, a sunscreen should be applied generously, which means about a teaspoon for the face, neck and décolletage.

If you are in Australia, use the SunSmart app, which will give you more precise details regarding the amount of sunscreen needed (based on the areas of skin exposed).

### *Believing that reapplying sunscreen will multiply its protective effect*

Reapplying sunscreen regularly might replace some of the product lost through sweating or friction. However, it will not extend the amount of time that you can safely stay under the sun for. Let me explain: if you usually start getting sunburnt after five minutes spent in the sun (like me!), a sunscreen with an SPF of 30 will only allow you to extend your daily sun exposure by up to two and a half hours (5 minutes x 30 = 150 minutes = 2.5 hours).

### *Thinking that a sunscreen can give you 100 per cent protection against UV radiation*

Even a broad spectrum sunscreen with the highest SPF never completely protects you against UV damage. Always remember that the best sun protection is to stay out of the sun!

When in the sun, always make sure to add to your sun protection by covering your skin with light-coloured clothes and by wearing a wide-brimmed hat and sunglasses (this is not only to prevent the eye contour from getting sun damaged, but the inside of your eyes too).

*Thinking that windows protect you against skin damage caused by*
*UV radiation*

Glass is able to block UVB radiation and prevent us from getting sunburnt. However, it cannot entirely shield us from UVAs (even if the glass has been treated).

If you live in a sunny place and are a regular car driver, have a look at your face in a mirror and compare the skin on both sides of your face: you are likely to notice more sun damage on the side that is the most exposed to the sun: the driver's side. So, to keep dark pigmentation marks and wrinkles at bay, use sunscreen even when you drive. Especially if you live in Australia!

*Thinking that a suntan makes you less susceptible to sun damage*

You do not need to get sunburnt for your skin to get sun damaged. In fact, a tan is also a sign of trauma, which indicates that your skin is trying to fight UV damage (mainly UVA radiation, the one that is responsible for the worst damage in your skin).

*If you really want a tan,*
*fake it and get one in a tube!*

---

## Choosing the right sunscreen

A lot of people shy away from using sunscreen as they find them too greasy or because they are afraid of the risk of adverse reactions such as skin irritation or breakouts. However, I cannot stress enough the importance of using sun protection products as an integral part of your skincare and as your best weapon against premature ageing. Choosing the product that suits you best may mean trying a few out before you find one that you really like.

# Sunscreen recommendations

The following sunscreens are well liked and tolerated by most of my clients:

## La Roche-Posay Anthelios XL SPF 50+ Extreme Fluid (Origin: France)

**Type:** Sunscreen with both physical and chemical sunscreen actions, very high broad spectrum UV protection.

**Note:** Anthelios XL SPF 50+ Extreme Fluid has a more runny consistency than most other 50+ sunscreens on the market. It feels very soothing on the skin and is recommended for normal to combination skin. This is a great choice for sensitive skin or skin prone to sun allergies.

## La Roche-Posay Anthelios XL SPF 50+ Melt-In Cream (Origin: France)

**Type:** Sunscreen with both physical and chemical sunscreen actions, very high broad spectrum UV protection.

**Note:** Anthelios XL SPF 50+ Melt-In Cream feels richer than its Extreme Fluid cousin but feels as gentle on the skin. This sunscreen is suitable for drier skin types as well as sensitive skin or skin prone to sun allergies.

## Sunsational Clear Sunscreen SPF 50+ (Origin: Australia)

**Type:** Chemical sunscreen, very high broad spectrum UV protection, four-hour water resistant.

**Note:** Clear Sunscreen SPF 50+ is a lightweight, non-clogging sunscreen with a sheer finish. It is very easy to apply and dries quickly. It can be used on all skin types and makes a good make-up base.

# Moisturiser with SPF product recommendation

If you cannot surpass your aversion for sunscreen, try this moisturiser with SPF as your next best option:

## O Cosmedics Mineral Pro SPF 30+ (Origin: Australia)

**Type:** Moisturiser with physical broad spectrum UV protection action.

**Note:** Mineral Pro SPF 30+ is a zinc oxide–based hydrator that contains some antioxidants and peptides for free-radical protection and skin repair. It is also available in a tinted formula.

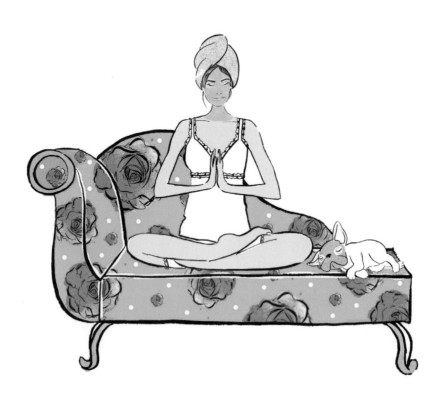

# CHAPTER 4

## USING A SERUM, EXFOLIATING AND MASKING YOUR SKIN

Have you mastered your basic daily skincare rituals that consists of cleansing, toning, moisturising and using sun protection? Are you ready to expand on your routine? Let's get into it!

# Using a serum

### The benefits of using a serum

Serums are designed to work on specific skin concerns such as dehydration, lines and wrinkles, pigmentation, skin irritation, skin congestion or breakouts.

### About serums

Traditionally, facial serums have a higher active ingredient content than face creams. They also tend to be more water-based, which makes them lighter and faster-absorbing into the skin. Serums can be used all over the face, neck and décolletage (as in the case of a hydrating serum) or more locally (for example on the the T-zone only when wanting to control excessive oiliness).

Many serums contain strong active ingredients. Please read the labels carefully and consult 'Key corrective active ingredients' in Chapter 2 for precautions and contraindications before use.

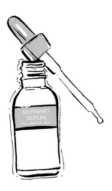

### How to use your serum

Most serums are meant to be used after cleansing and toning, and before the application of a moisturiser.

Apply your serum in the same way you apply your moisturiser: place a little serum onto your fingertips, usually half a pea to a pea-sized amount for the entire face and neck, and a little more for the décolletage. Press your fingertips onto your cheeks, forehead, chin, neck and décolletage. Spread over the skin until all areas are covered.

Of course, if you are only using your serum on a localised area (for instance the cheeks or the nose), adjust the amount of serum to the area of skin that you are wanting to treat.

**EXPERT TIPS**

Always check the manufacturer's instructions as some serums are meant to be used at night when skin repair is at its peak, or to avoid the risk of your skin becoming sensitised by some ingredients that should not be exposed to the sun (this is the case of some vitamin A and fruit acid–based serums).

Sometimes, some serums are also supposed to be mixed with other products such as a moisturising cream or even a mask. So, again, it is always wise to check your product packaging for specific usage instructions.

## A common misconception about serums

*Thinking that you always have to use a cream on top of a serum*

Sometimes, you can just use a facial serum by itself. It just depends on your skin type!

## Choosing the right serum

A serum should be selected according to the skin concern that you want to address (and not based on its fancy name!). Always think about what you want to achieve and then question how a particular serum is going to do what you want it to do: which active ingredients does this serum contain? Are these ingredients best suited for the job of hydration, exfoliation, brightening, etc.?

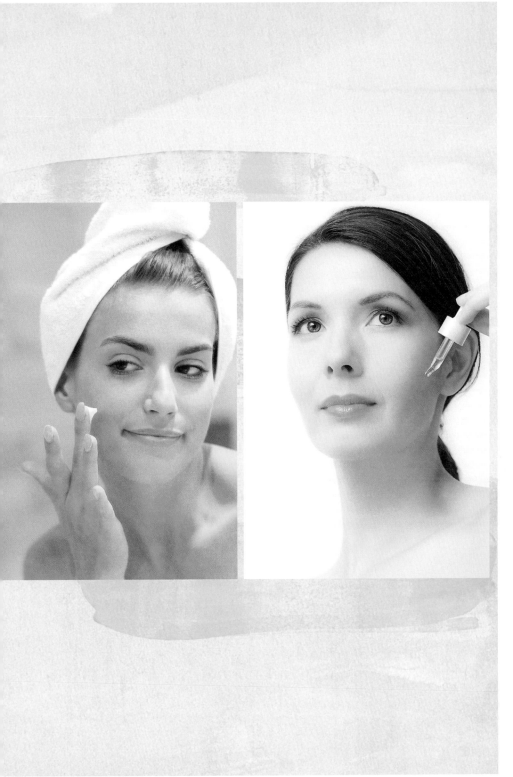

# Late teens and twenties serum product recommendations

Are you getting zits? If you are, the use of serums can help you in your fight against breakouts. However, make sure NOT to use products that are too harsh: you might be breaking out, but there is no need to punish your skin for it! You and your complexion need tender loving care and a skin-friendly serum that can work its magic on your congestion and your blemishes.

## Skin Juice Liquid Tri Active Clearing Serum (Origin: Australia)

This serum is a great alternative to harsh and drying benzoyl peroxide–based products. Its ingredients (alpha and beta hydroxy acids and some botanical extracts) help clear the skin by targeting the three key issues that are associated with breakouts and acne: excessive oiliness, clogged pores and inflammation-causing bacteria. **Liquid Tri Active Clearing Serum** can be used all over the face or on areas of concern, alone or under a moisturiser.

## Sircuit Skin Cosmeceuticals Fixzit Blemish Drying Serum (Origin: USA)

**Fixzit Blemish Drying Serum** should be used sparingly as this is a potent serum that is NOT designed to be used all over the face, but rather as a localised spot treatment for your blemishes. It contains a powerful blend of fruit acids and retinol to exfoliate, unclog, purify and speed the healing of blemishes. A very effective spot treatment.

# Thirties serum product recommendations

Are you looking tired and in need of a boost? Are you starting to notice some unevenness in your skin colouring? Are some sun spots beginning to appear on your skin? It seems like you may need some brightening up. Here it comes, in an easy-to-use serum form!

## Skin Juice Shine Resurfacing Serum (Origin: Australia)

I like to use this serum alone, once to three times a week when I feel like my skin needs a little tonic. With a gentle blend of alpha hydroxy acids, a natural whitening complex (Whitami) and some papain, **Shine Resurfacing Serum** boosts and illuminates the complexion. It also works very well at preventing congestion and breakouts by assisting the skin's natural renewal process. Perfect!

## Sircuit Skin Cosmeceuticals Sircuit Weapon 10% Vitamin C Therapy Serum (Origin: USA)

This is more than just a plain skin-brightening vitamin C serum: **Sircuit Weapon** is pumped up with powerful active ingredients including hyaluronic acid for hydration (*oui!*), resveratrol for free-radical protection, squalane to nourish and protect as well as copper peptides to rejuvenate. *J'adore!* Can be used alone or under a moisturiser.

# Forties serum product recommendations

In your forties, lines and wrinkles are likely to have become your primary skin concern. Your tools: a cosmeceutical fruit-acid serum to refine your skin at night time AND a cosmeceutical moisture-binding serum to boost skin hydration to be applied in the morning.

## Image Skincare Ageless Total Anti-Aging Serum (Origin: USA)

This serum uses a unique delivery system (vectorise technology) that prolongs the release of alpha hydroxy acids, peptides, antioxidants and apple stem cells which all combine to smooth the epidermis and promote skin repair and protection. This means that once applied to the skin, **Ageless Total Anti-Aging Serum** works for longer (up to 48 hours) to improve your skin tone and texture. To be used under a moisturiser.

## Image Skincare Ageless Total Pure Hyaluronic Filler (Origin: USA)

I would describe this serum as a free-radical fighting and skin-plumping serum, all-in-one. **Ageless Total Pure Hyaluronic Filler** is definitely one of the products that I would take to a desert island with me since it gives such impressive results. You can mix it with your moisturiser or you can use it straight onto your skin before applying your cream. I prefer the second option because it allows you to specifically target your fine lines and wrinkles. This is a fantastic product with a very well-suited name!

# Fifties and beyond serum product recommendations

As we get older, our skin may become more reactive: this is due to the fact that it tends to be thinner and drier than before (less oil means less protection). In addition, our immune system is less reactive and slower to come to the defence of our skin. These factors contribute to making our largest organ more vulnerable to irritation and in greater need of soothing, especially if you are currently going through menopause and are experiencing hot flushes. Your skin does not need to feel like an industrial strength radiant heater!

## Uskincare Sensitive Rescue Serum (Origin: Australia)

Being aloe vera based, this serum is extremely calming. It contains some of the most healing botanicals, including pure essential oil from German chamomile. This essential oil would have to be one of my favourites: such a soothing elixir with such an amazing colour: a deep blue, which gives **Sensitive Rescue Serum** its unique tinge. A great serum to use every time your skin needs cooling and healing. This product may also help alleviate some of the skin inflammation associated with acne, eczema, rosacea or even sunburn (in this case, you can refrigerate prior to using as this will give you a more intense cooling sensation. NOT that your skin would EVER get sun damaged, would it?!).

## Sircuit Skin Cosmeceuticals Nineoneone Calming Serum (Origin: USA)

This calming serum works very well on my rosy cheeks (I am prone to redness which seems to show more after a glass of Bordeaux, but I am quite fine with champagne, *merci* for asking). **Nineoneone** has such an impressive ingredient list! Essential fatty acids, peptides, witch hazel, aloe vera, allantoin . . . you name it! It also contains 'soft focus' powder to visually enhance the complexion (it does have a nice blurring effect on redness, fine lines and wrinkles).

# Exfoliating your skin

## The benefits of using an exfoliant

Exfoliation is necessary to boost desquamation – the natural shedding of dead skin cells from the surface of the skin. Regular exfoliation makes your skin texture more even and softer. It also increases the efficacy of skincare products as they are able to penetrate more deeply into the skin. All this leads to a more vibrant and younger appearance. Minimising the build-up of excess dead skin cells on the surface of the skin by exfoliating regularly can also reduce the likelihood of getting breakouts.

Many exfoliants contain strong active ingredients. Please read the labels carefully and consult 'Key corrective active ingredients' in Chapter 2 for precautions and contraindications before use.

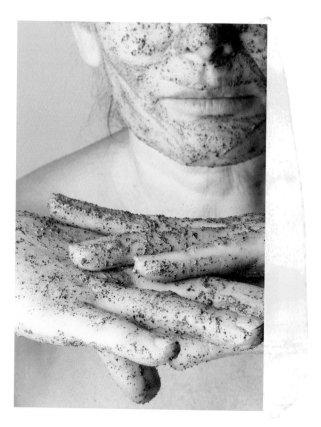

# About exfoliants

Exfoliants basically all fall into two distinct categories: mechanical and chemical exfoliants.

## Mechanical exfoliants: scrubs and gommage exfoliants

Mechanical exfoliants are abrasives that work by physically removing some of the dead skin cells that are part of the skin surface. Once applied to the skin, they need to be manually rubbed on for their action to occur. They can be used on all skin types except those that are highly sensitive or those affected by severe acne (the action of physically working this type of exfoliant on the skin would be too stimulating and would also increase the chance of spreading the infection).

### Scrubs:

Scrubs are the most common exfoliants on the market. Their exfoliating action can be based on various exfoliating particles such as ground apricot kernels, walnut shell powder, diatomaceous earth, jojoba beads or microbeads.

### Gommages:

Gommage products have become a little old fashioned. This is probably because they can be quite messy to use and they are also more time-consuming to work with (applied like a mask onto dry skin, a gommage should be left to dry for a few minutes before it is carefully rubbed off the skin, hence the extra time required).

Did you know . . . ? The term 'gommage' means 'erasing' in French. It refers to the action of rubbing away the dead skin cells from the skin surface.

## Chemical exfoliants: enzymes and fruit acids

Chemical exfoliants work by chemically dissolving the bonds that hold the dead skin cells of the skin's outer layer together. These may come in the forms of cleansers, toners, serums, creams, masks or peels.

### Enzymatic exfoliants:

Enzyme-based exfoliants contain fruit enzymes such as papain (from papaya) or bromelain (from pineapple). They can be used on all skin types and are especially well suited to fine and sensitive skin.

### Fruit acid exfoliants:

- *Glycolic and lactic acid (alpha hydroxy acids or AHAs)*
  Glycolic acid can be used on all skin types. However, it can be more irritating and drying to the skin than lactic acid (due to its smaller molecular size, which allows for a deeper skin penetration). For this reason, lactic acid is better suited to sensitive, dry and dehydrated complexions.

- *Salicylic acid (beta hydroxy acid or BHA)*
  Oil-soluble by nature (like all BHAs), salicylic acid is able to penetrate inside hair follicles where it clears the build-up of dead skin cells that contribute to skin congestion and breakouts. It also has an anti-bacterial and anti-inflammatory action on the skin which is helpful when treating acne.

Retinol and exfoliation

Although the common side effects of using topical vitamin A can resemble those associated with the use of some fruit acid exfoliants (can include skin dryness, peeling, irritation and discomfort), retinol is not classified as a chemical exfoliant but as a cell-renewal booster. Retinol can be used in conjunction with chemical exfoliants (or with gentle physical ones). As an example of a product that contains both retinol and chemical exfoliants, see my reference to *Image Skincare Ageless Total Repair Crème* in the 'Minimising the appearance of fine lines and wrinkles' section in Chapter 5.

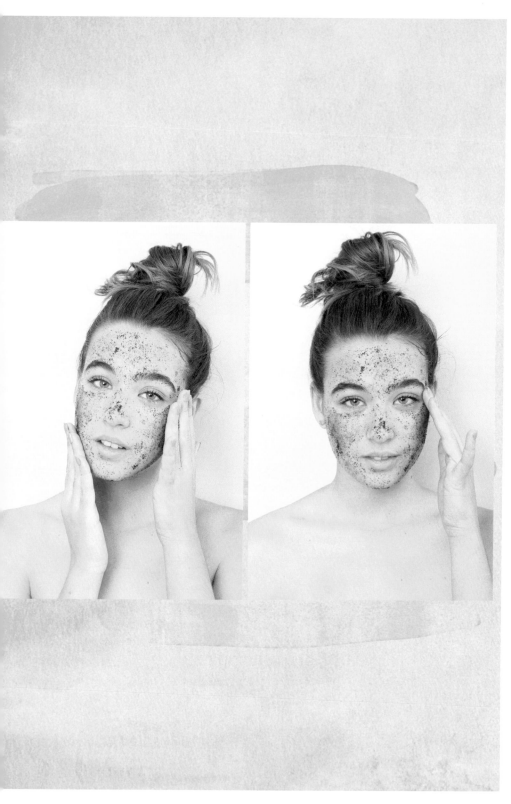

## How to use your exfoliant

Exfoliants should always be used on cleansed skin (this is why I am not a big fan of exfoliating cleansers and always recommend using separate and stand-alone cleansing and exfoliating products). Exfoliating once or twice a week is usually plenty.

### *Scrubs*

After cleansing your skin, apply a small amount of scrub to your face, neck and décolletage using wet fingertips (avoid the eye area). Gently massage for a few minutes using circular movements. Persist a little longer on congested areas such as your nose and chin. Rinse off well with lukewarm water.

> **EXPERT TIPS**
>
> Choose a scrub with small and rounded exfoliating particles so as to avoid skin damage (irregular particles can create microscopic tears in the skin).
>
> It is a good idea to test a scrub on the skin of your inner forearm first: massage in a small amount of product and make sure that it does not feel too harsh or scratchy.
>
> If your scrub feels too harsh for you, mix it with a little cleansing milk or cleansing cream before using (but still cleanse your skin first before you exfoliate). This simple step will soften its action.
>
> You can also control the action of a scrub by adjusting the amount of pressure used when massaging it onto your skin: the heavier your hand pressure, the stronger the action of your scrub will be. No need to go hard for a scrub to do its job!

## Gommages

After cleansing your skin, pat it dry with a tissue. Apply a small amount of gommage to your face, neck and décolletage using dry fingertips (avoid the eye area). Leave on for a few minutes. With the index and middle fingers of one hand, form a V and place on your skin for support. With the fingertips of your other hand, gently rub the supported area to remove the gommage. Move to the next area of skin to be exfoliated and repeat the process until the exfoliation is complete. Rinse your skin well with lukewarm water.

**EXPERT TIPS**

Be sure to remove your gommage over a basin as removal can be quite messy.

Do not wait until your gommage is totally dry before beginning your exfoliation as this will make its removal much harder and could potentially irritate your skin. If you have allowed the product to over-dry, use a slightly damp fibrella to help rub it off the skin.

## Chemical exfoliants

Chemical exfoliants, both enzymatic and fruit acid–based, should be applied on clean and dry skin (avoid the eye area). Follow the manufacturer's instructions: these are unique to every chemical exfoliant (some of them must be removed from the skin, others should be left on).

**EXPERT TIP**

ALWAYS follow the manufacturer's instructions as some chemical exfoliants can be quite potent and have the potential to cause damage to your skin if not used appropriately.

# A common exfoliating mistake

## Over-exfoliating your skin

The current beauty trend is to put faces through a continuous refining boot camp with a view to revealing younger and more 'perfect' skin: scrubbing, brushing, peeling, resurfacing . . . let's do it all and as often as we can! This philosophy does NOT work, believe me! I see so much skin damage done by excessive exfoliation: a lot of stripped, dehydrated, irritated, over-thinned, damaged and prematurely aged faces, all needing to be healed, repaired and nurtured. The fact that this compulsive practice is being promoted by some of my own industry colleagues really saddens me and makes me question their motivation: do they really care about people's skin or are they more concerned with flogging products and selling treatments? Remember that harsh and constant interfering with the normal functioning of our skin is detrimental to it and that we need some of these dead skin cells and surface oils: they are essential to the integrity, good health and good looks of our skin. Let's work with our skin, not against it!

> ### EXPERT TIPS
>
> Check the active ingredients of every skincare product that you use to evaluate how much and how often you are actually refining your skin. Apart from your mechanical or chemical exfoliating products that are clearly marketed as 'exfoliants', you could be using other refining products on your skin without realising it: AHAs, BHAs and vitamin A could be hidden in some or all of your other skincare products, especially if they are cosmeceutical ones.
>
> Go easy on cosmeceutical-strength products as some of them can be quite potent and sometimes harsh. Monitor your skin and adjust your exfoliating routine accordingly: if your skin feels irritated and sore, stop using the offending product and give your skin time to repair itself.

# Choosing the right exfoliant

*Mechanical exfoliant or chemical exfoliant?*

We know how good exfoliating can be for the skin. However, the wrong choice of exfoliant may be more detrimental than beneficial. So, always keep in mind that everyone's skin is unique and that what works for a friend might not work for you. As mentioned previously, various exfoliating products suit different skin types and conditions. Your lifestyle should also be taken into consideration before making your selection.

## EXPERT TIPS

Avoid using a scrub or gommage if you are suffering from acne as the mechanical action of exfoliation may contribute to the worsening of your condition. Choose an enzymatic or a fruit acid–based exfoliant instead.

Do not use a scrub or gommage if your skin is very thin or lacks elasticity as you could be causing damage to it, including broken capillaries and bruising. Choose an enzymatic exfoliant instead.

Do not use a strong chemical exfoliant such as a peel in summer if you are planning to spend the whole day outdoors, as it makes your skin more susceptible to sun damage and pigmentation. Always keep in mind that even the best sun protection product will never protect you 100 per cent against harmful UV rays.

If your skin type and condition permit, I suggest alternating between physical and chemical exfoliants for the most complete, rounded treatment: a chemical exfoliant to loosen up the attachments between your dead skin cells and a physical exfoliant to take them away. But do not use them together: leave a few days between both types of exfoliations.

# Late teens and twenties exfoliant product recommendations

Exfoliation is an important step in your skincare routine at this age as it helps reduce pore congestion and overall build-up of dead skin cells from the surface of your skin. Also think of regular exfoliation as an extra preventative measure against pimples.

## Skin Juice Pulp Clarifying Cleansing Paste (Origin: Australia)

This is a deep cleansing cream that I like to use as an exfoliant (on previously cleansed skin). It is perfect for oily or combination skin that has a tendency to congestion and breakouts. It combines the gentle absorbing actions of white clay together with the exfoliating powers of salicylic acid and bamboo granules to leave your skin cleaner, softer and healthier.

## Uskincare Bamboo Polish (Origin: Australia)

**Bamboo Polish** is a refreshing scrub that is packed with antioxidants. Bamboo grounds exfoliate and refine the pores while ginkgo and ginseng extracts are used to invigorate and revitalise the skin. A polishing treatment for the face, to leave it nice and smooth and lovely!

# Thirties exfoliant product recommendations

As you get into your thirties, you may start to notice some unevenness in your skin colouring. Your complexion may even look dull and lifeless. Do not despair: a little exfoliation will perk you up. There is no better enlivening treatment than gently massaging an exfoliant over your face. So, off to the bathroom to exfoliate!

## Sircuit Skin Cosmeceuticals Sir Activ Zeolite Invigorating Scrub (Origin: USA)

This is a powerful physical exfoliant that works thanks to the presence of jojoba beads, diatomaceous earth and cranberry seed powder. Its deep skin cleansing action is assisted by zeolites (which are dirt- and impurity-drawing minerals). **Sir Activ** suits skin that is prone to congestion and that lacks a little lustre. You can use it up to twice a week (try not to overuse just because you like its lovely cranberry pink colour and cranberry scent!).

## Dermalogica Daily Microfoliant (Origin: USA)

This universally well-known exfoliating powder has a real brightening effect on the skin, not only thanks to its enzymatic action on the skin but also from an added grapefruit and licorice complex. This is why it works well at reducing skin congestion and improving skin tone. It is a very similar product to **Indeed Laboratories Facial Powdered Exfoliator,** as described in the 'Fifties and beyond' section. Both products are marketed for all skin types. However, I find **Daily Microfoliant** more suited to oily and combination skin (since it contains salicylic acid, the exfoliating agent of choice for oilier complexions). Although its name suggests otherwise, there is no need to use **Daily Microfoliant** every day: two to three times a week should suffice.

# Forties exfoliant product recommendations

In your forties you are likely to invest more into beauty products. However, there is not much point in spending money on expensive treatment serums and creams if you are not regularly exfoliating your skin. Exfoliation is an efficient way to give your skin a helping hand by boosting the absorption of active ingredients so you get the best results out of your skincare products.

## Phytomer Vegetal Exfoliant with Natural Enzymes (Origin: France)

For a product that is meant to stay on your skin for a short time (five to ten minutes), **Vegetal Exfoliant with Natural Enzymes** really delivers! It does act like a real skin treatment since it gives your skin an enzymatic exfoliation (from papain) and a hydrating boost (from laminaria digitata seaweed). All in one! It is definitely the kind of skincare product that every time-poor woman should have (and use!).

## Gernetic Ger Peel (Origin: France)

This scrub is superb: its creamy texture and the choice of microcapsules as exfoliating agents both allow for a uniform and safe exfoliation. **Ger Peel** leaves your skin extremely smooth, refined and polished. Oh, and I should add that a little of this product goes a long way (a tube should last you a full year).

# Fifties and beyond exfoliant product recommendations

In your fifties and beyond, there is a real risk of damaging your skin by using the wrong exfoliating products. As your skin matures, it tends to thin and it becomes more fragile. Hence the importance of choosing gentle products that will not harm you. You just want your skin to look refreshed, not irritated or bruised!

## Institut Esthederm Osmoclean Gentle Deep Pore Cleanser (Origin: France)

This deep cleansing product gives all the benefits of a gommage without its downside. It leaves the skin incredibly smooth and purified, it is non-messy (it does not leave any residue behind), and it is recommended for all skin types including delicate and older complexions as well as those affected by acne (since it does not need to be rubbed off the skin, just lightly massaged).

## Indeed Laboratories Facial Powdered Exfoliator (Origin: Canada)

This is a truly impressive facial exfoliant that can be used on any skin type since it is gentle and non-stripping. It contains both physical and chemical exfoliating agents: bromelain to enzymatically exfoliate and a soft blend of bamboo extracts and rice bran powder to gently buff away your excess dead skin cells. A little hyaluronic acid has also been added for hydration. You mix a little **Facial Powdered Exfoliator** with water, massage onto the skin for about 60 seconds and rinse off. Quick and easy!

# Using a facial mask

## The benefits of facial masking

I am a huge fan of facial masking! In fact, using a facial mask is a bit of a tradition among French women. I grew up watching the two generations of women before me applying all sorts of mask concoctions on their skin. Applied regularly (once or twice a week), facial masks can make a noticeable difference to the way your skin looks, improving it significantly. Depending on their ingredients, masks can achieve a broad variety of effects such as purifying, exfoliating, soothing, hydrating, firming, whitening or nourishing. I cannot stress enough the beneficial effects of masks on the skin!

## About facial masks

Here is an overview of some key active ingredients found in facial masks, together with their properties.

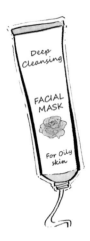

### Purifying

- Clay is definitely the ingredient of choice for deep cleansing masks.
- Clay has the ability to draw out impurities from the skin. For this reason, clay-based masks can be beneficial for skin that is prone to breaking out or developing blackheads.
- Various clays have different degrees of potency: kaolin is one of the most gentle, and Fuller's earth the strongest and the most stimulating of clays.
- I like to use French clay because of its high degree of effectiveness and also for its versatility (and not because I am French!). French clay comes in different levels of strength (drawing ability) so it can suit even the most sensitive skin.

## Exfoliating

Enzymes and fruit acids can be added to a mask to create a skin-refining effect.

• **Enzymes:** as seen previously in the section on exfoliation, the most common enzymes used are papain (from papaya) and bromelain (from pineapple). If your skin is sensitive and reactive, choose an enzyme-based exfoliating mask over a fruit acid–based one: enzymatic masks tend to be more gentle.

• **Fruit acids:** some exfoliating masks can contain AHAs, which work well on sun damaged, mature, dry or congested skin. Others contain BHAs and are more suited to oily skin.

## Soothing

Calming mask ingredients may include aloe vera, manuka honey or chamomile.

• Aloe vera gel is not only soothing, it also has a good hydrating effect.

• Manuka honey is renowned for its natural healing properties. It is also anti-bacterial and for this reason can be helpful to skin affected by acne.

• Chamomile (sometimes listed as azulene) can benefit highly reactive skins thanks to its strong anti-inflammatory effect, which can help reduce skin redness.

**EXPERT TIP**

If you would like your soothing mask to be even more soothing on your red cheeks, cool it down slightly before use (leave it for one hour in your refrigerator). This will cause your blood capillaries to contract and will help temporarily reduce the amount of redness in your skin.

## Firming

Firming masks create a temporary lifting effect on the skin thanks to the action of ingredients such as albumen and wheat protein.

• Albumen (obtained from eggs) is a protein that creates a firming film on the skin and also helps with skin hydration.

• Wheat protein has similar firming properties to albumen.

**EXPERT TIP**

For a skin pick-me-up effect, use a firming mask just before you go out. Don't worry, the effect will last long enough so you do not have to feel like Cinderella at midnight!

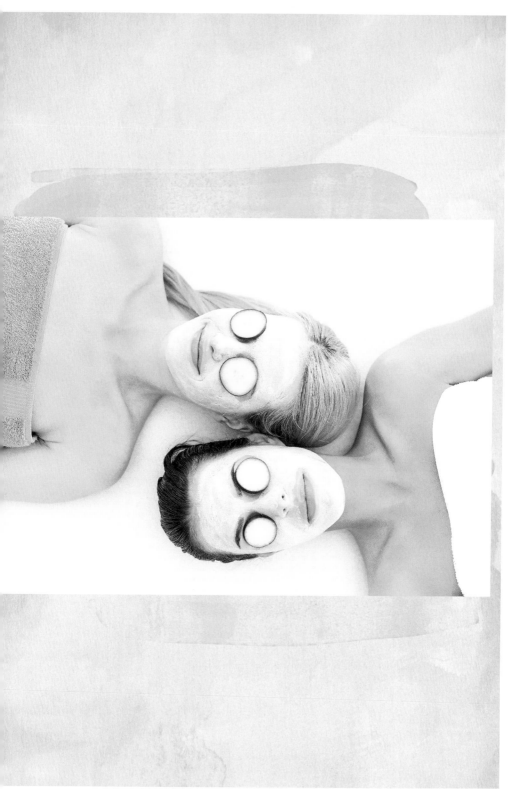

## Hydrating

Moisturising masks are likely to include ingredients such as glycerin, jojoba oil or seaweed extracts.

• Glycerin has a strong water-binding ability and helps make the skin look smoother.

• Jojoba oil acts as a fantastic moisturiser as it prevents excessive water loss from the skin.

• Seaweed possesses highly hydrating and remineralising properties. (A decade ago I spent a week in the French coastal city of Saint-Malo in Brittany where I immersed myself in the world of thalassotherapy, a spa industry that utilises the healing virtues of seawater and seaweed on the skin and body. So therapeutic that even French doctors recognise their benefits!)

**EXPERT TIP**

To boost the efficacy of your hydrating mask, apply your mask and then have a warm bath: instead of becoming evaporated, the water lost from your skin (as a result of your body trying to regulate its temperature) will remain under the mask and be used to further re-hydrate the surface layer of your skin. Warning: not too much champagne please (it is dehydrating).

## Whitening

Whitening masks do not make your skin white! They are designed to fade skin pigmentation and brighten the skin thanks to ingredients such as kojic acid and licorice extract.

- Kojic acid and licorice extract work by inhibiting tyrosinase, the enzyme involved in the production of melanin, our dark skin pigment.

> **EXPERT TIP**
>
> Using a whitening mask alone is unlikely to make your pigmentation disappear totally: you need to add a good lightening product (see the 'Reducing dark pigmentation marks' section in Chapter 5). However, it will always brighten and enliven tired skin.

## Nourishing

Nourishing masks contain ingredients such as avocado oil, macadamia oil or shea butter.

- Avocado oil is an easily absorbed, nutrient-rich oil that helps protect and repair dry or mature skin.
- Macadamia oil is light in texture but loaded with essential fatty acids that help lubricate the skin and restore its barrier function.
- Shea butter is a deeply rejuvenating ingredient that comes from the nut of the karite tree.

> **EXPERT TIP**
>
> To create a more intensive effect from your nourishing mask, leave it on your skin overnight (and cleanse your skin in the morning as normal). To do this without leaving a mess on your pillow, apply a thin layer of the mask and massage it into your skin for about 10 to 15 seconds or until it has completely absorbed. You can do this once or twice a week. *Bonne nuit!*

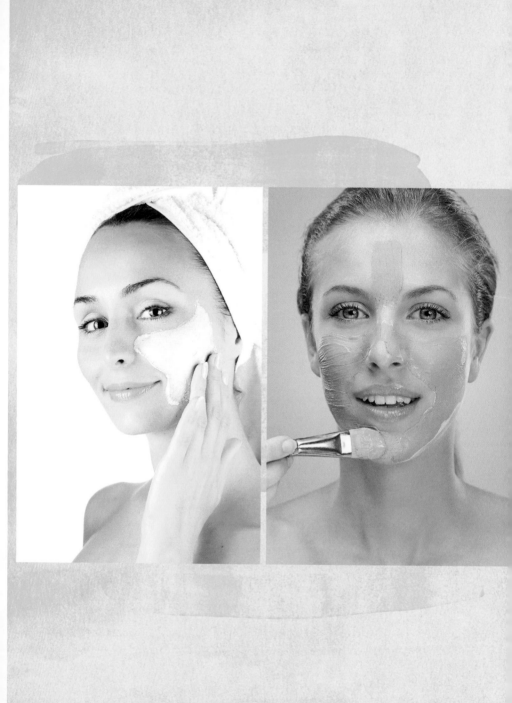

## How to use your facial mask

A facial mask should always be applied on clean skin. Whether you use your fingertips or a mask brush (a medium-sized synthetic foundation blending brush works well), apply your chosen mask to the entire face, neck and décolletage. Leave on the skin for the required amount of time (follow the manufacturer's instructions, especially when using an exfoliating mask). Remove with plenty of lukewarm water. Follow by moisturising your skin.

**EXPERT TIP**

Please note that facial masks should not be used too close to the eye area. For the delicate eye contour, choose a mask especially designed to be used on that area, or use a thick layer of your eye cream.

## A common misconception about using a mask

*Thinking that you have not got the time to use one*

Once you have applied your mask, you do not have to stay still until it is ready to be removed (although the option of lying down with your feet up and a good book should always be the preferred option!). If you are too busy for a pause, do what you have to do while the mask is working on your skin: some household chores, preparing a report, making phone calls . . . multi-tasking beauty! Not ideal relaxation time but better than missing out entirely.

## Choosing the right facial mask

Choose your mask in accordance to your skin type and condition. What are you wanting to treat? Do you want to purify, exfoliate, soothe, hydrate, firm, whiten or nourish your skin? Of course, you can use two different masks on various parts of your skin. For instance, you can use a purifying clay-based mask on your T-zone and a hydrating mask over the rest of your face, neck and décolletage.

# Late teens and twenties mask recommendations

At this age, your skin is likely to be clogged and breakouts may be frequent. If you do get pimples, always keep in mind that picking at them NEVER makes them go away quicker! On the contrary, each time you interfere with your blemishes, you are disturbing the natural healing process of your skin, which means that your blemishes will stay on for longer. Not to mention the risk of permanent scarring. So hands off and go and mask your face instead!

## Palmer's Cocoa Butter Formula Purifying Enzyme Mask (Origin: Australia)

This is a thick dual-action mask that combines the drawing and purifying action of kaolin clay with the gentle exfoliating effect of papaya enzyme. **Purifying Enzyme Mask** leaves your skin cleansed and soft without stripping it. Although indications on the packaging specify that you can use it up to three times a week, once or twice a week should suffice. You can also use this mask as a spot treatment on your blemishes.

## Antipodes Aura Manuka Honey Mask (Origin: New Zealand)

This mask feels extremely healing and medicinal on the skin. I like the fact that it is hydrating and that it leaves the skin soothed. It is recommended for blemish-prone and/or dehydrated skin but could be used by anyone wanting a gentle cleansing and refreshing skin treatment.

# Thirties mask recommendations

In your thirties, the visible signs of fatigue caused by too many late nights or a too-hectic lifestyle become harder to hide. But do not despair since a good facial mask can give your skin a true beauty flash effect. And, of course, masking is also a great way to practise ESC (Extreme Self-Care) which we all need in our life!

## Bliss Triple Oxygen Instant Energizing Mask (Origin: Switzerland)

This innovative mask feels like a brightening spa facial at home. A great product to use if you are time poor as it achieves its mission in minutes. It comes out of its container as a light cream that you massage onto your clean, damp skin. It soon starts frothing and quickly transforms into a dense foam which you then rinse off your skin. **Triple Oxygen Instant Energizing Mask** is ideal for normal, combination and oily skin that is in need of enlivenment. **Tip:** I would not recommend this mask for dry, sensitive or acne-prone skin as it would be too stimulating on these skin types. Do not use exfoliating or refining products on the same day, as this is a potent mask.

## Image Skincare Vital C Hydrating Enzyme Masque (Origin: USA)

This fresh and creamy enzyme-based mask gently encourages the removal of excess dead skin cells while feeding your epidermis a powerful cocktail of antioxidants (vitamins A, C and E). This results in a softer, plumper and revived complexion. **Vital C Hydrating Enzyme Masque** can be used on all skin types. A gentle exfoliant and a hydrating mask all in one: how handy!

# Forties mask recommendations

In your forties, masking is a must! I will never get tired of promoting the many benefits of facial masking. 'Mask, mask, mask!', I tell my lovely clients all day. Sometimes, it takes quite a bit of nagging on my part to make them commit to this extra home-care step. But it is all worth it in the end. I love to see their reaction once they start to witness the changes in their skin. And then, I tell them: 'You see? I told you so! *Très bien!*

## Gernetic Hydra Ger (Origin: France)

You will particularly benefit from using this creamy white kaolin clay–based mask if you have combination or oily skin that is also dehydrated. As soon as **Hydra Ger** begins to set, it starts to gently exfoliate and purify the skin without depleting its moisture levels. This mask is definitely far more hydrating than your traditional green clay mask.

## Sircuit Skin Cosmeceuticals Cool Lychee Wa Intensely Hydrating Mask (Origin: USA)

This deeply hydrating mask does feel very cooling on the skin. It also has a strong antioxidant effect due to its rich free-radical fighting ingredients (lychee, goji berries, mangosteen and green tea). **Cool Lychee Wa**: a mask with a playful name but with a serious mission to rejuvenate all skin types!

# Fifties and beyond mask recommendations

At this tender age, your skin sometimes feels that it can never get enough moisture in. This is when masks become extremely handy! Indeed, a good hydrating mask can supplement the action of your moisturising serums and creams. Together with a good water intake and lots of fruits and vegetables: winning!

## Avène Soothing Moisture Mask (Origin: France)

Recommended for dry or sensitive skin, this white and creamy mask eventually absorbs into your skin to leave it nourished, plump and calm. You can leave **Soothing Moisture Mask** on overnight and you could also use it as a skin conditioning treatment (instead of a moisturiser) in case you find yourself on one of those long flights to Paris. *Bon voyage!*

## Skin Juice Vanilla + Honey Moisture Massage Mask (Origin: Australia)

This is a rich mask with a beautiful texture. It is full of lovely fats and oils that nourish and protect the skin. Shea butter, mango butter, cocoa butter, safflower oil . . . the list is too long! **Vanilla + Honey Moisture Massage Mask** can also be left on the skin overnight (it absorbs into the skin once you massage it in), and you just need to rinse it off in the morning. You can also use this product to perform my healing massage routine (see Chapter 8).

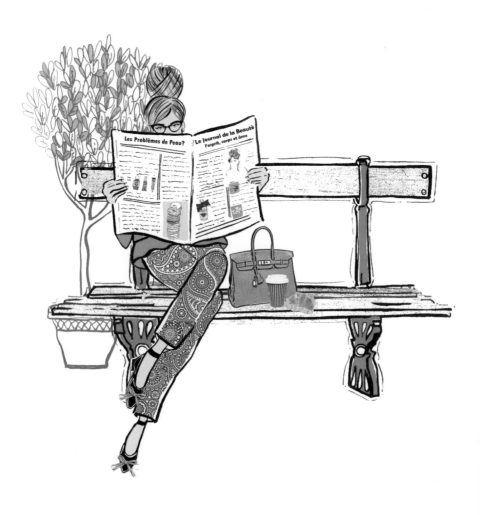

# CHAPTER 5

## DEALING WITH YOUR SKIN PROBLEMS

# Minimising the appearance of fine lines and wrinkles

Fine lines and wrinkles will ALWAYS look more pronounced on dry and dehydrated skin, so the secret lies in keeping your skin's oil and water levels well adjusted . . . along with a few other little blurring secrets!

## Action plan

- **Have a weekly lactic acid peel.** This will not only help get rid of the excess dead skin cells that can make your skin look dull and tired, it will also help make your skin look plumper and more hydrated. I like **Sircuit Skin Cosmeceuticals Mocha Loca Chocolate Lactic Acid Peel**, which is a great chocolate-scented lactic peel that is suitable for all skin types.

- **Alternatively, you can use a retinol-based cream to help reveal younger-looking skin and stimulate the production of collagen in your skin.** I like **Image Skincare Ageless Total Repair Crème.** This is a potent refining night treatment cream that contains a 20 per cent blend of glycolic acid and retinol. It is suitable for all skin types. However, do not use if your skin is sensitised. Always introduce slowly.

- **If you have dry skin, give it its daily dose of nourishment in the form of richer cleansers and creams that contain plenty of emollient-type ingredients** (those lovely fats and oils!). See Chapter 3 for more details about moisturisers.

- **Boost your general hydration levels by drinking lots of water and eating plenty of fruits and vegetables.** Plant foods have a high water content and have the added bonus of being able to powerfully combat skin ageing due to their strong antioxidants properties.

- If you are specifically concerned about fine lines and wrinkles around the eyes, try **Image Skincare Ageless Total Eye Lift Crème.** This eye cream contains a mild blend of glycolic acid and retinol to gently resurface the skin. Apply at night and combine with a more hydrating eye cream such as **Image Skincare The Max Stem Cell Eye Crème.**

- **Incorporate hyaluronic acid–based products into your daily skincare regime.** Hyaluronic acid is a fantastic cosmetic active ingredient since it has a great ability to bind moisture to the skin by holding up to 1000 times its weight in water: this results in plumper, smoother skin and visibly diminished fine lines and wrinkles (*oui, merci!*).

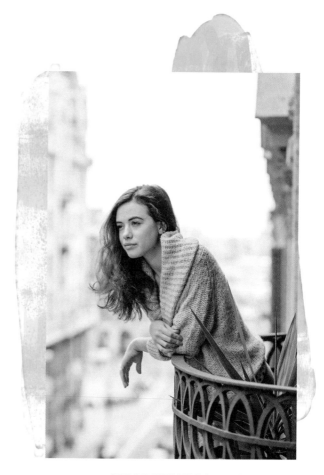

I am particularly impressed by the three hyaluronic acid–based products that I mention below as I have seen spectacular results on myself and my clients from using them.

Just follow these steps:

## Step 1

After cleansing and toning, apply a few drops of **Image Skincare Ageless Total Pure Hyaluronic Filler** directly onto the lines and wrinkles that you are wanting to minimise and massage into the skin for a few seconds until absorbed. This product has a very fitting name and it is by far the best skin plumping serum I have tried. Keep using your serum daily as it has a cumulative effect on the skin.

## Step 2

Follow with a moisturiser (see 'Moisturising your skin' in Chapter 3). If your skin is dehydrated all over, you can also mix a few extra drops of **Ageless Total Pure Hyaluronic Filler** into your moisturiser. You can stop here or choose to continue with Step 3.

## Step 3 (optional)

Add a little light-reflecting effect to your look by using either of these hyaluronic acid–based complexion-perfecting products:

- **Embryolisse Artist Secret Complexion Illuminating Veil BB Cream** (Origin: France). This product best suits normal to oilier skin types. It gives a good medium coverage with a matt finish. I find this tinted cream particularly suited to skins that have a tendency of breaking out since it contains gently exfoliating fruit acids (BB stands for 'blemish balm').
- **Auriège Paris Lift CC Cream** (Origin: France). This cream is more hydrating than **Artist Secret Complexion Illuminating Veil BB Cream** and more suitable for normal to dry skin types. It gives a slightly lighter coverage but has a more dewy and light-reflecting finish (CC stands for 'colour correcting').
  (**Note:** Both of these products can be used instead of a moisturiser or as a primer. Both products come in one single shade that adapts to most skin colours, although dark skin tones will need to use a darker foundation colour on top.)

# Minimising the appearance of 'open pores'

I prefer to use the term 'enlarged pore' to refer to an 'open pore' as this is more correct. Although the term 'open pore' is widely used, a pore cannot open or close since it does not have a muscle! Genetics have a lot to do with the size of our pores, and so does ageing (our pores tend to become more apparent with age due to a decrease in our skin density). While you cannot totally eliminate enlarged pores, you can certainly minimise their appearance by working on refining your skin. In French, we say *affiner le grain de la peau* (which translates as: 'to refine the grain of the skin').

## Pore-minimising products

- To promote exfoliation, use an AHA-based serum. I like **Image Skincare Ageless Total Anti-Aging Serum**.
- Perform a weekly enzyme peel at home. I find that **Epicure Cosmeceuticals Enzyme Peel: Pumpkin** works very well at resurfacing the skin. If your skin is too sensitive for a resurfacing peel, try a more gentle exfoliating approach by using an enzymatic exfoliant such as **Dermalogica Daily Microfoliant** two to three times a week.
- Treat and camouflage your pores with a good BB cream. The very best I have tried is **Embryolisse Artist Secret Complexion Illuminating Veil BB Cream**, which suits a normal to oilier skin type and gives a matt finish. As mentioned previously, you can use this tinted product alone, or on top of a moisturiser for extra hydration. It has the added advantage of acting as a pore refiner by gently exfoliating your skin thanks to its mild fruit-acid blend. (Please note: do not use Artist Secret Complexion Illuminating Veil BB Cream straight after a fruit-acid peel as this product contains a mild AHA blend.)
- If you prefer an uncoloured product rather than a tinted BB cream, opt for **By Terry Hyaluronic Hydra-Primer Colorless Hydra-Filler**: applied on top of your moisturiser, this primer will still give you a matt finish but will look invisible on your skin (no tint). You may then follow with a foundation.
- Read Chapter 6 to discover Victoria Martin's make-up secrets, which will complete your look.

# Reducing under-eye dark circles and puffiness

The reasons why we may develop under-eye dark circles and puffiness can be associated with genetics (people of African or Indian descent are more prone to this problem), our state of health and our lifestyle. The ageing process can also be a factor: the blood capillaries of the eye contour tend to become more apparent as our skin becomes thinner, and puffiness increases as our circulation starts to work less effectively.

## Action plan

- If you suffer from hay fever or chronic sinus infections, make sure to seek medical treatment for these conditions first as they can cause dark circles and puffiness.
- Make adjustments to your lifestyle so as to improve your level of general health: diarise regular breaks from work, get some fresh air, go to bed earlier, eat a balanced diet and be mindful of not taking on too much (say 'no' more often!).
- Discourage fluid retention by drinking more water, by reducing your alcohol and salt intake and by being more active (even a gentle walk every day encourages the body's circulation).
- Apply a cool compress on your eyes to help decongest the eye contour: dampen a small towel with refrigerated water and place on your eyes for 10 to 15 minutes. Follow with the application of an eye care product.
- Use a specific eye product to help relieve congestion and brighten the eye area. As mentioned in Chapter 3, I have been getting excellent results with **Epicure Cosmeceuticals Skin Firming Eye Serum.** This eye serum contains a good blend of cutting-edge active ingredients including ones that specifically target dark circles and puffiness (green-coffee extract, Eyeseryl, Haloxyl and Bioskinup).
- Read Chapter 6 to discover Victoria Martin's make-up tips, including her fabulous under-eye concealing secrets.

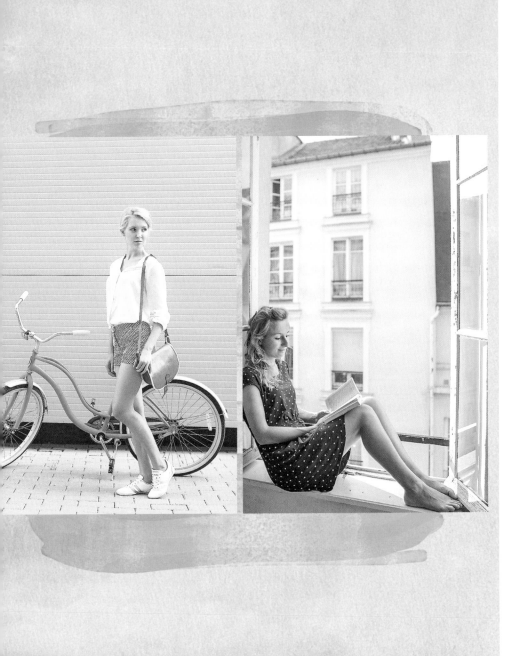

# Getting rid of blackheads, whiteheads and milia

As mentioned before, blackheads are little plugs made of dead skin cells and hardened sebum that obstruct the opening of a hair follicle. They look black because they have oxidised once in contact with the air.

Whiteheads are similar in composition to blackheads but are much less obvious since they are partially covered by some skin cells (which prevents them from turning black).

Milia are different altogether: they are tough little cysts made of dead skin cells that are trapped within the skin. As they are harder to remove, they must be professionally lanced in order to be freed from the skin.

## Removal

Contrary to what some skincare companies would want you to believe, there is not a cream out there that can dissolve blackheads, whiteheads or milia: you need to physically remove them.

I would discourage DIY extractions as it is very easy to damage your skin by applying too much force and using the wrong extraction technique. It is best to leave your blackheads *et al.* alone and book yourself in for a professional facial that includes extractions.

**Important:** prior to making your appointment, make sure to select a practice that has high standards of cleanliness and hygiene.

You can prepare your skin for a professional extraction session by hydrating and exfoliating your skin prior to your facial appointment:

## Step 1

Two to three weeks prior to seeing your facialist, start using (if you are not already) a hyaluronic acid–based serum every night under your moisturiser. This simple step will make your skin more supple and extractions much easier to perform. And this makes them much more tolerable for you! **Image Skincare Ageless Total Pure Hyaluronic Filler** or **Indeed Laboratories Hydraluron** work well on all skin types (you can use either one of these serums any time you want extra skin hydration, whether your skin is prone to congestion or not).

## Step 2

Three days prior to your professional extraction session, exfoliate your skin with a gentle chemical exfoliant such as **Phytomer Vegetal Exfoliant with Natural Enzymes** or **Image Skincare Vital C Hydrating Enzyme Masque,** which is a little stronger. Both products are suitable for all skin types and have the added advantage of leaving your complexion well hydrated. Use them as you would any mask, leave on the skin for five to ten minutes, rinse off well and apply your moisturiser.

## Preventing blackheads, whiteheads and milia

You can delay and sometimes even prevent some blackheads, whiteheads and milia from re-forming by making sure that you maintain a regular skincare regime that includes exfoliation.

If you are prone to skin congestion, avoid using skincare products that are too oily as these could have a comedogenic effect on your skin. This means that they could clog your pores and therefore encourage the formation of blackheads and whiteheads.

*Working at keeping your pores decongested will also reduce the likelihood of getting acne breakouts.*

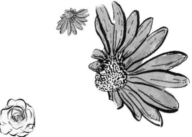

# Managing acne

Suffering from acne can be extremely distressing, especially if all your attempts at finding the right skincare products have failed. But it is wise to avoid anyone (or any product) who promises instant results: this is totally unrealistic as your skin needs time to heal properly (in my experience, you need three to six months minimum, depending on the severity of your condition).

If you are suffering from severe acne, you are probably under the care of a dermatologist, who might have prescribed a specific treatment for you. Please note that I am not advocating ditching your doctor or dermatologist here! I am simply sharing with you some practical information and tips that I have found to be helpful in managing and improving acne.

**Important:** Please note that you should always consult with your medical professional first before introducing new skincare products. You want to make sure that they will be compatible with the medical treatment that you have been given (especially if you are on Roaccutane as this drug makes your skin extremely dry, fragile and sensitised).

## Action plan

- **Make sure to be extremely hygienic when handling your skin:** wash your hands before and after touching your face and use single-use disposable items as much as possible. I recommend using fibrellas to help remove products from your skin (see 'Cleansing your skin' in Chapter 3). And of course, don't use cleansing brushes, sponges or loofahs on your skin.
- **Change your pillow case often** (every day if you can).
- **Wash your make-up brushes every few days** with mild antiseptic liquid soap (invest in a second set of brushes so you always have a clean and dry one).
- **Choose your haircare products carefully** (favour natural organic brands). Wash your hair often with a mild shampoo. Do not use too much hair styling product and do not put any on your skin. Also, keep your hair off your face.
- **Find a facialist who can guide you and support you** (alongside your dermatologist) on your journey to clear skin. What you need is a clear treatment plan, honesty and encouragement along the way.
- **Be extra gentle with your skin.** Avoid rubbing or massaging the affected area as this would worsen your skin condition and irritate your skin further. The only form of massage that can assist in clearing acne is a professional lymphatic massage (check if your facialist is trained in lymphatic drainage techniques).

- **Resist squeezing your pimples:** remember that the more you pick at your pimples, the more likely you are to spread the infection and make your acne worse. Also keep in mind that interfering with the natural healing process of the skin only causes pimples to linger, not to mention the risk of permanent scarring and hyperpigmentation of the skin.
- **Swap your conventional foundation for a mineral powder.** Most make-up products tend to make acne worse, so make sure to use high quality make-up brands that have been especially created for problem skin. I personally like **Mineralogie.** Their make-up products are made with high quality ingredients and are non-clogging. They also give you a very good and natural coverage.
- **Treat your skin in a holistic way.** Read this book in its entirety and make some lifestyle changes.
- **Pay particular attention to the link between your diet and the behaviour of your skin.** Do you find that some foods can make your acne breakouts worse? Based on my experience as a facialist, I can report that acne tends to get worse when people indulge in a diet rich in sugar, dairy, wheat and processed foods, hence the importance of eating fresh, wholesome food that does not come out of a packet. Your local farmers' market is always a better option than the supermarket!
- **Consult a naturopath.** This might not only help you improve your general health but also identify some nutritional intolerances that could have an impact on your skin. Last year, a client of mine with inflamed acne found out from a naturopath that she was fructose-intolerant. Once she eliminated fructose from her diet her skin quickly became much calmer and, with a good skincare regime, her breakouts drastically lessened over a few months. She is now clear of acne.

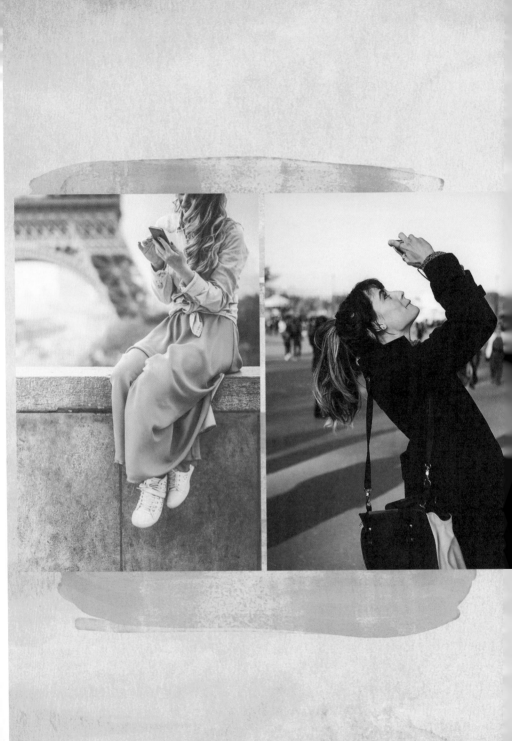

## Acne-fighting products
## (also suitable for skin experiencing occasional breakouts)

In order to successfully treat acne the products you use must address these four key points simultaneously, *without* stripping or irritating your skin:

1. Remove excess oiliness and impurities.
2. Decongest blocked follicles.
3. Reduce skin inflammation.
4. Keep your skin hydrated.

You can do this by using a non-stripping cleanser, a light moisturiser and a good exfoliating salicylic acid serum. Every acne case is different and should be assessed individually. However, I consistently have a high level of success with the following products. Please note that you do not need to have acne to use these products: I do also recommend these to clients with congested skin or skin that experiences any occasional/localised breakout.

### Image Skincare Ormedic Balancing Facial Cleanser (Origin: USA)

This is an effective yet gentle cleansing gel that also removes make-up well. It helps control oiliness without stripping or dehydrating the skin, and it has a calming effect. To be used morning and night.

### Image Skincare Vital C Hydrating Anti-Aging Serum (Origin: USA)

This hydrating product is usually well tolerated by acneic skin. It gives a matt, non-greasy finish, which is quite welcome by anyone who has oily skin. To be used in the morning and/or at night on clean skin, not only as a light-textured moisturiser but also as a great skin repairing, antioxidant product.

### Sircuit Skin Cosmeceuticals Sircuit Agent (Origin: USA)

Sircuit Agent contains a blend of alpha and beta hydroxy acids, some lemon peel extract and some apple stem cells that give exfoliating, decongesting, antimicrobial, anti-inflammatory, brightening and repairing properties to this serum. This product gives AMAZING results on acneic skin and is definitely well worth the expense. It is much more gentle on the skin than most acne products available on the market (it does not strip the skin). It can be used all over the face (except the eye area) or locally, on affected areas only. Use at night on clean skin.

# Managing rosacea

These days, I see more and more women with rosacea, a distinctive disorder that shows as skin redness (from mild to severe), periodic flushing and small acne-like breakouts. Although the cause of rosacea has not been established for sure, genetics and skin colour are major contributing factors in its development: the fairer your skin is, the more chance you have of developing rosacea. And as there is no cure for rosacea, the emphasis of your skincare should be on minimising its flare-ups and reducing the chance of them getting worse.

## Action plan

- **Treat your skin in a holistic way.** You cannot successfully control rosacea by relying on skincare products alone and, as with acne, your approach should be all-encompassing so as to give yourself a better chance of tackling this skin condition. Read this book in its entirety and make some lifestyle changes.

- **Make it a priority to reduce stress in your life.** Based on the conversations I have had with my past and present clients who suffer from rosacea, I do note that, in a lot of cases, the onset of the condition correlates with periods of extreme emotional stress (such as starting a highly stressful job, a relationship breakup or the cancer diagnosis of a loved one). Obviously, a lot of stressful situations are out of our control. However, what we can do is to implement some self-preserving strategies that can help us when tough life challenges come our way (see Chapter 7).

- **Pay more attention to your feelings.** My philosophy is that we all need to acknowledge what we feel since suppressing our emotions has a negative impact on our bodies and can show on our skin (this is definitely the case for rosacea). There is no such thing as a negative emotion: even anger can be useful as it can be a way of finding out what frustrates us and what we wish to let go of in our lives.

- **Pay particular attention to your diet** and avoid elements that may trigger rosacea flare-ups: the worst culprits tend to be sugar, spicy foods, dairy foods and stimulants such as coffee, chocolate and alcohol, since they all can have an inflammatory effect on the body.

- **Avoid temperature extremes,** such as harsh weather conditions (if you can), and hot baths and showers.

- **Avoid sun exposure.** Protect your skin from UV radiation by using a broad spectrum sunscreen with a high SPF (don't forget your hat and sunglasses!).

- **Avoid any harsh in-salon treatments.** When I treat a client with rosacea, I perform a simplified facial consisting of a gentle cleanse, a very mild exfoliation (it might take quite a few sessions to strengthen the skin before an exfoliation can be performed), some lymphatic massage and the application of a calming mask. And of course, I always end with an application of sunscreen if it is a daytime appointment.

## Rosacea-friendly products

I am reluctant to recommend specific skincare products here as, unfortunately, rosacea being such a reactive and complex condition, what might work for one person's skin could be irritating to another. However, the general skincare recommendations I can make are:

- Stay away from heavily perfumed skincare or products that are strong on essential oils as these can irritate the skin further.
- A skincare range that seems to be particularly well tolerated by a lot of people with compromised skin (including those affected by rosacea) is **La Roche-Posay Toleriane**. But again, it is really a case of trial and error with rosacea.
- Keep your skincare routine extremely simple: cleanse, moisturise and use sun protection.
- Tread lightly: avoid too much friction and use light pressure on your skin.

*If you are fair skinned, reduce your chances of developing rosacea by following my above-mentioned tips BEFORE the condition occurs.*

# Reducing dark pigmentation marks (hyperpigmentation)

Hyperpigmentation is commonly seen in my new homeland, Australia, since one of its main causes is exposure to sunlight. UV radiation can play havoc with our melanocytes – the skin cells that produce the pigment melanin. Sometimes, it causes a disorganised increase in the production of melanin, which shows as darker patches on the skin. Other causes of hyperpigmentation include some medications (including the contraceptive pill), fragrances in skincare, some hormonal disorders, pregnancy and also the natural ageing process of the skin.

The first thing to do is obviously to establish the cause of your hyperpigmentation. If it is caused by medication, talk to your doctor to try and find an alternative. If the culprit is a fragranced or essential oil–based cosmetic product, stop using it!

In any case, protect your skin against UV radiation as exposure to sunlight has a darkening effect on pigmentation (there is no point in trying to lighten your skin with specific serums and creams if you keep exposing it to the sun and if you do not wear sunscreen!). Use a broad spectrum sunscreen with a high SPF (at least 30) and be sun smart. This is particularly important if you are pregnant or taking the contraceptive pill, or if you are using fruit acid or vitamin A–based products, which increase your skin's sensitivity to the sun. (For more details and tips, see 'Using sun protection' in Chapter 3.)

## Hyperpigmentation-fighting products

To date, the most effective skin lightening agent is hydroquinone but, as it can have strong side effects (these include skin irritation and even skin discolouration), it is worthwhile trying milder and better-tolerated products first.

Most cosmetic products targeting hyperpigmentation combine exfoliating ingredients (chemical exfoliants) with other active ingredients that have tyrosinase-inhibiting properties. These tyrosinase inhibitors are known to be able to help reduce the action of tyrosinase, the enzyme needed to produce melanin.

Some of my clients have been getting great results with **Sircuit Skin Cosmeceuticals Brilliance Fading Serum**, a skin-lightening serum that combines the actions of lactic acid, lemon peel extract and Phenylethyl Resorcinol (one of the newer cosmetic active ingredients used for its fading and antioxidant properties).

I have also witnessed some noticeable reduction in hyperpigmentation with the combined action of two **Gernetic** products: **Skin Clair Concentrate** to exfoliate and **Skin Clair Nutritive Cream** to treat and hydrate. Both contain a botanical complex that includes mulberry and licorice extracts (well-known tyrosinase inhibitors). The concentrate should be applied under the cream as a spot treatment for darker patches.

One way to boost the efficacy of your lightening serum is to use it in conjunction with lactic acid or vitamin A. **Sircuit Skin Cosmeceuticals Double Trouble 5% L-Lactic Pomegranate Acai Peel** contains both ingredients. It is a home-care lactic acid peel that specifically targets hyperpigmentation. It is to be used once a week and to be followed by a moisturising cream (wait a day or two after this peel to use your lightening serum).

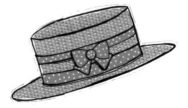

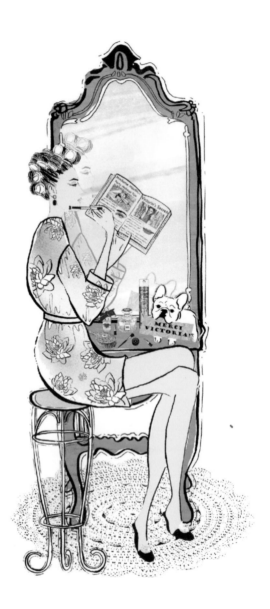

# CHAPTER 6

## USEFUL
## MAKE-UP TIPS

*with Victoria Martin*

Like most French women, I believe that make-up should be used to enhance your natural features and not as a camouflaging agent. However, achieving a polished make-up look does require a certain level of knowledge and skill. So, here comes Victoria Martin! Victoria is a leading make-up artist and one of my beautiful clients. Here she is going to divulge some of her invaluable expert tips and secrets. And now, over to you, Victoria!

## What are your priming secrets?

Priming the skin before make-up application means you are preparing the skin, ensuring it is clean, well hydrated and smooth. For some people, a simple application of moisturiser will suffice, and certainly that is what most people did before the arrival of specific 'priming' products. Always try before you buy and see how the product works in your current routine. At the end of the day, it is really dependent on your skin type, what feels comfortable and the effect you want to achieve. Some of my favourite primers are as follows:

### For dry/dehydrated skin
I like **Embryolisse Lait-Crème Concentré**, it gives amazing instant hydration and a beautiful smooth base to work with.

### For normal skin
**By Terry Hyaluronic Hydra-Primer Colorless Hydra-Filler** works really well to fill in any fine lines or pores and gives a matt finish on which to apply your foundation product. It gives a plump, hydrated look for the whole day.

### For oily skin
I recommend **Hourglass Veil Mineral Primer SPF 15**. This is quite a liquid consistency when first applied, but then dries to a smooth, almost powdery finish because it is oil free. It is also water resistant and has an SPF of 15.

### For a glowy make-up look
Try the **Tom Ford Illuminating Primer** as it has an ultra-fine micro shimmer which gives a luminous sheen to the skin. Great when used underneath your foundation or, for more glow, mix the two together and then apply.

# What is your top make-up tip for appearing younger?

## Less is more

As women get older, the tendency is to wear heavier, stronger make-up in an attempt to cover/conceal/hide signs of ageing. In fact, heavy foundation and concealer will only make you look older. Instead, ensure your skin is well hydrated and opt for a sheer foundation or tinted moisturiser, and gently define your features for the best results. By this I mean: don't go overboard with make-up; focus on your favourite features and enhance them. For example, if everyone always tells you your lips are fabulous then make lip colour your 'thing'. Alternatively, if you have beautiful sparkly eyes then play them up with lots of mascara and eyeliner. However, always make sure you have balance – take time to step back from the mirror and look at your face overall. In addition, investing in good quality brushes will help you instantly and give a more refined and professional finish.

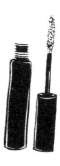

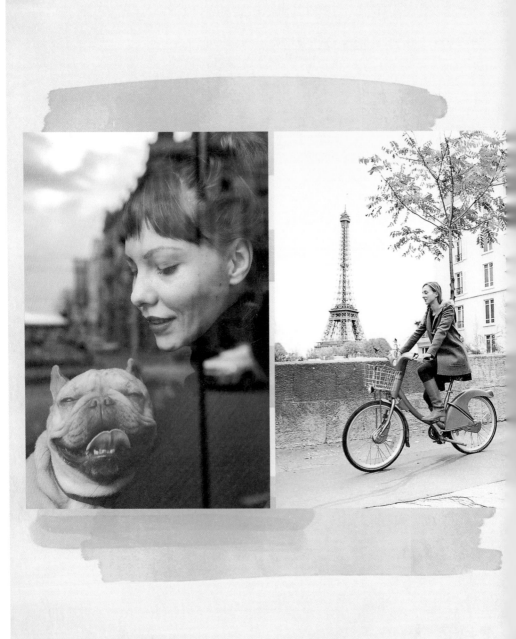

# What is the best way to conceal pimples?

There is a common misconception out there that make-up can totally conceal a blemish. Here is the truth: make-up can even out the colour, or hide any redness associated with a pimple, but it will not cover the texture. By this I mean: if you have a pimple that is raised or irritated, make-up cannot take this away, and if you cover your pimple in make-up it really won't help the healing process. If you can manage it, my best tip would be to let the skin recover and heal without any extra products on top. However, if you have a special event you need to attend or a hot date (and pimples always seem to appear exactly when you don't want them to) there are ways to conceal it:

1. The first step is to reduce swelling. I like to wrap a few ice cubes in a tea towel or face cloth and gently apply to the area for a few minutes.
2. If the area is dry or flaky, gently hydrate with a light moisturiser.
3. Apply your normal primer and foundation first. It will probably cover more than you expect.
4. Now take a matt concealer that matches your skin tone (I like **Clé de Peau Beauté**) and, using a small synthetic concealer brush, apply the product to the blemish and surrounding area in a soft pressing motion. Refrain from rubbing or irritating the area further. In the area around the blemish, sheer out the concealer until it disappears. If you think you still need more coverage, allow the product to set for a few minutes and have a look in natural light before you add another layer.
5. To hold the concealer in place you will need a small amount of powder. Go very light on this as you don't want to highlight the texture of the blemish. Use a delicate tapping motion with a small natural-hair brush like an eye shadow brush.

For more serious acne or blemishes my favourite product is **Vichy Dermablend**. It gives a high coverage (it needs to be used sparingly) but it will cover blemishes, scratches and scars.

# What is the best way to cover dark circles under your eyes?

The best way to go about this is to first hydrate the under-eye area with a very light eye cream and allow it to absorb a little. The next step is to assess whether you need a corrector to neutralise the colour. If you feel like you have tones of blue or green you will probably need a corrector. My favourite is the **Bobbi Brown Corrector** which comes in a variety of shades. Using a flat, synthetic brush, apply the corrector to wherever you see that dark shadow – normally it is in the inner corner of the eye. Then pat and press it in with your ring finger. Then you will need to apply the **Bobbi Brown Creamy Concealer** – to lift and brighten the corrector shade – with a similar process: apply where you need it with the brush and then tap in with your finger. The final step is a light dusting of powder to set the products you have applied.

If you feel this process is too much for you then an alternative is to use a more liquid formula such as the **Ellis Faas Concealer**, which comes in a pen applicator. This will probably feel lighter, but will not cover the darkness as effectively as a cream. It is an issue of personal taste and depends on how 'polished' you want to look.

# What is the best way to deal with droopy eyelids?

Unfortunately droopy eyelids are another part of the ageing process. However, here are a few insider tricks that can help the situation.

- **Refrain from applying mascara to your bottom lashes;** this will only drag the eye down. Instead, curl your top eyelashes really well with the **Shu Uemura Eyelash Curler** and then apply several coats of mascara.
- **Keep your eyeliner to the top lashline only,** and as close to the roots of the lashes as possible. Always make sure your eyeliner pencil is nice and sharp before you apply. A blunt pencil is only going to make your life harder and won't give any precision.
- **If you do decide to wear eye shadow, avoid frosted eye shadows** – they will exaggerate the appearance of fine lines and wrinkles. The only exception to this is using just a little shimmer on the inner corner of the eye to open it out. A soft champagne shade usually works well.

# What is the best way to make a wrinkle less apparent?

No make-up product will ever make wrinkles or lines disappear. But the best answer to this is to minimise the use of oil-free products and powder.

First off, ensure your skincare is hydrating and plumping – and this goes for your foundation products too. There are many oil-free foundations on the market so always check the bottle and the fine print before you buy. An oil-free foundation will be long lasting but it will generally be quite matt, which accentuates fine lines. So always opt for a hydrating, lightweight foundation formula which blends in to your skin and gives a bit of glow and youth.

When it comes to powder, if you are very concerned with wrinkles I would suggest you skip it altogether. If you have oily tendencies in your T-zone, then a very light dusting of finely milled powder applied to only that area with a powder brush will do the trick. Avoid using a powder puff to apply powder as it will give a heavy coverage and look very drying. My favourite is the **By Terry Hyaluronic Hydra-Powder** which is ultrafine and colourless. It feels very smooth and light on the skin due to its silica microbeads.

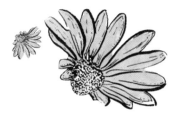

# Late teens and twenties make-up essentials

Your twenties are a time of experimentation, so don't be afraid to try out bold colours or a smoky eye. However, I would still recommend letting your natural beauty show through. At this age, your skin will be youthful and glowing so make the most of it and select a lightweight foundation or even a tinted moisturiser.

## NARS Lipstick

NARS offers a beautiful range of lip colours, in various textures (sheer, semi-matt and satin) for every mood. Experiment with a hot pink like 'Schiap' or channel your inner Audrey Hepburn with the delicate pastel 'Roman Holiday'.

## MAC Face and Body Foundation

This cult foundation is ideal for a girl in her twenties since it gives light to medium coverage and is easily applied using fingers. It gives a beautiful, healthy glow to the skin without ever looking heavy. My best advice when using this product is to work quickly, in sections around the face, pressing it into the skin.

## Clé de Peau Beauté Concealer

You may still suffer from the odd blemish during your twenties so having a creamy concealer on hand will be useful. This formula from Clé de Peau Beauté is smooth and easy to blend and looks just as good if you're using it on bare skin or in partnership with a foundation/tinted moisturiser.

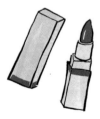

# Thirties make-up essentials

Women in their thirties start to grow in confidence and generally feel more comfortable in their own skin. This goes hand-in-hand with make-up. So, let that confidence guide you in your choices.

## Red lipstick

I am a firm believer that every woman should own a red lipstick, and in your thirties it is the perfect pick-me-up. The lipstick doesn't necessarily have to be opaque and bright, there are other red options out there for every woman. For first-time users, go for a sheer moisturising formula like **Chanel Rouge Coco Shine in 'Rebelle' (63)**. A step up from that is **Clarins Joli Rouge Lipstick in 'Clarins Red' (716)**. It is a hydrating but pigmented true red. Finally, if you're feeling brave, you can't go past the iconic **'Ruby Woo' by MAC**, an opaque matt red that will turn heads. My biggest tip with red lipstick is to use a matching red lip liner to prevent bleeding or feathering.

## Urban Decay Naked Eyeshadow Palette

During your thirties, I would recommend starting to invest in high-quality products for your make-up kit, and this palette is a great place to start. It is universally flattering, with 12 neutral eye shadow shades that can take you from day to night and everything in between. The colours come in a good variety of shimmer and matt options ranging from champagne tones to mid browns and bronze to greys and plums. The shade 'Darkhorse' is a standout as it is a perfect mocha brown with a hint of shimmer. You could use it as part of a smoky eye application or, if you are fairer skinned, as eyeliner pressed in to the lashes.

## Bobbi Brown Corrector and Creamy Concealer

At this time in your life, you're likely to be working harder, and with more responsibilities you might notice your under-eyes suffer. These products can help to even out that area of the face. It works in two stages: first the Corrector eliminates the blue/green shadow and then the Creamy Concealer is used to lift and brighten. The formula is smooth and doesn't cake.

# Forties make-up essentials

Once your forties hit, you will begin to see some changes in your skin, blotchiness, age spots or redness. You may also notice some lines and wrinkles. Using make-up in a careful and selective manner can help combat some of these signs of ageing.

### Clarins Beauty Flash Balm

This is a real favourite and it delivers an instant lift to lacklustre or dull skin. It is ideal as a make-up primer under your foundation, or can even be used on its own for a clean, radiant complexion. To apply, smooth it on (a pea-sized amount for the whole face) rather than rub it in.

### Bobbi Brown Long-Wear Cream Shadow

This eye shadow formula stays put all day and doesn't crease or accentuate fine lines. My favourite colours in the range are 'Shore', a neutral cream which gives a fresh look for most Caucasian women. 'Suede' has a bit more depth and I would describe it as a creamy tan brown, great for all eye colours. For night-time, 'Velvet Plum' is a warm bronze plum colour with a metallic finish.

### By Terry Crayon Khol Terrybly

At this stage the lashline will start to look less defined, so use a soft eyeliner pencil such as this one from By Terry to give more intensity. Dot it in between the lashes first, then join the dots along the upper lashline. Then go in with an eyeliner brush or your little finger to soften the line. Make sure you go right to the inner corner. If you stop halfway or two-thirds of the way it will look unfinished and give the impression that your eyelashes stop growing at that point. Generally, I would recommend lining just the upper lashline since it makes your eyes look bigger and more open. Stay away from lining inside the waterline; this will definitely make your eyes look smaller.

# Fifties and beyond make-up essentials

Less is definitely more once you get to fifty and above. Choose hydrating, light formulas, and a hint of colour on the lips and cheeks will work wonders.

## Kevyn Aucoin The Volume Mascara

Eyelashes get sparser and lighter with age, so my best recommendation is **The Volume Mascara by Kevyn Aucoin**. The lash-building fibres thicken and define to emphasise the lashes and it is extremely long wearing. Apply more than five coats over previously curled lashes to get beautiful definition.

## Lipstick Queen Invisible Lip Liner

I would definitely suggest continuing to use lip colour for this age as it can really lift the face. However, you will find that the line of the lips may become less distinct and lip colour might feather or bleed. To fight this, use a clear silicone-based lip liner like the one from Lipstick Queen to trace the shape that you want to create before you apply your lipstick. Also be wary of dark or metallic lip colours as they will make the lips look thinner. My tip is to use something hydrating or with a touch of gloss to give the impression of fuller lips.

## Anastasia Beverly Hills Brow Wiz

By this stage your eyebrows have probably become quite thin and sparse so by filling them in you can give your face more shape and ultimately look more polished. The Brow Wiz is a fine pencil with a wind-up tip on one end and a spoolie brush (mascara brush) on the other that allows you to imitate the appearance of tiny hairs for a fuller brow. Always pick a colour that is one shade lighter than your hair colour, so that it looks totally natural.

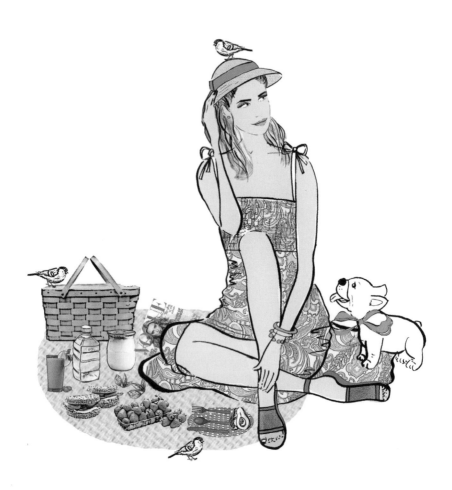

# CHAPTER 7

## SKIN-FRIENDLY
## LIFESTYLE

# Living the 'skin-friendly' lifestyle means reducing stress in your life

Stress is not always a bad thing, it just depends on how much of it we experience in our lives. In small amounts, it can be a good motivator to do well and achieve. For instance, it can encourage us to study before an exam or to prepare for an important work presentation. But prolonged exposure to stressful situations is harmful to us. When we are experiencing stress, our body switches to fight-or-flight mode – a built-in survival mechanism that redirects the flow of blood to the heart and muscles, at the expense of our digestive system and our skin. When we get stressed too often, our skin becomes chronically starved of nutrients and oxygen, and this makes it more susceptible to ageing.

Right! But how do you reduce stress when life gets crazy and when stressful events occur? The only way we can minimise the negative effects of unwanted stress is to make a conscious effort to take control of your life as much as possible.

## My suggestions for minimising stress

### Accept your life for what it is right now

Life can throw some real challenges at us, good and bad! In hard times, it is easy to feel like a victim of our own existence and to wish that our life were not the way it is. Unfortunately, this attitude does not serve us very well as it adds to our stress by fuelling frustration and hopelessness. It is always best to accept whatever happens to us and learn from every life situation.

> **MY TIP**
>
> Keep a gratitude diary: every day, write down at least three to five things for which you are grateful. This simple action really helps you to see the glass as half full rather than half empty, even when life gets tough! Personally, I like to do this first thing in the morning as it puts me in a positive mindset for the whole day.

## Set clear boundaries

As a woman, it is very easy to take on too much and, as a consequence, to lose all notion of life balance. Between our personal and professional life, so many often competing demands can be put on us! This is why it is essential to be clear and honest with ourselves about what we truly can and want to do. When we do not set limits around what we can handle, we not only increase our stress but we usually feel resentful too. This is not helpful!

**MY TIP**

Practise saying no without feeling guilty. And if you decline to do something, do not try and justify yourself. You have the right to say NO!

## Get inspiration from others

When stress takes over our life, when we feel overwhelmed and exhausted, words from others can be a terrific source of help and inspiration.

**MY TIP**

Subscribe to blogs that empower you to live a more balanced and authentic life (and cancel the others!). I personally love reading the comforting words of Leo Babauta, the person behind zenhabits.net, a blog about simplifying your life that is currently ranked in the top 25 out of the zillions of blogs out there in the world. Leo shares his own life lessons with refreshing honesty, and covers topics such as health, fitness, mindfulness and happiness.

## Make meditation a consistent part of your lifestyle

Meditation is very helpful in reducing stress and negative emotions. Personally, I believe that the regular practice of meditation allows me to manage my time better as it gives me more focus and a better sense of what my true priorities are. And this makes me feel less overwhelmed by the busyness of my life.

> **MY TIP**
>
> You do not have to be seated for hours in the lotus position to meditate effectively! You can reach a meditative state by simply going for a short walk in nature or by sitting alone in a quiet space for five or ten minutes. Take a few long deep breaths, relax, and enjoy being in the moment. What works for me is taking my two dogs (Marcel and Lily) to the park: the sheer fact of being among nature really gets me into the zone.

## Commit to exercising regularly

Apart from its obvious health benefits, exercise has an advantageous effect on our endocrine (hormonal) system and leads to the release of 'feel good' endorphins. This leads to healthier and more radiant looking skin.

> **MY TIP**
>
> Choose a sporting activity that you truly enjoy so it does not become a chore that causes you to feel more stressed. I personally love Pilates as it makes me feel really balanced and better equipped to deal with life demands. And I love walking to.

## Do something that you love

Making the time to indulge in something that you love doing can help to counteract the negative impact of stress by adding passion and spark to your life. It also keeps your spirit alive and joyful while preventing you from seeing life as 'all too hard'.

**MY TIP**

Ask yourself: 'What am I passionate about?' 'What do I love doing?' Whether it is cooking, spending time with your pets, writing, etc., diarise some time for your passion every week.

*Do something that makes you happy!*

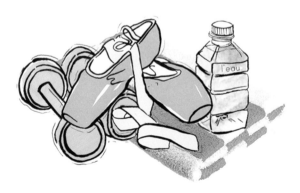

# Living the 'skin-friendly' lifestyle means getting enough beauty sleep

Our skin needs resting! It is during sleep that our body (including our skin) regenerates the most. When we do not get adequate sleep, our skin suffers and can age more rapidly.

## My suggestions for a good night's sleep:

### Avoid caffeine

Caffeine can affect people differently. But for most of us, the effect will be a decrease in the quality of our sleep, or even a total loss of sleep.

**MY TIPS**

Look for the hidden caffeine in foods and drinks. Caffeine is not only present in coffee, it is also in cola-based soft drinks, energy drinks, tea and chocolate. Have some chamomille tea instead since it is so soothing and calming.

### Have a light dinner

Have you ever noticed how eating too much at night can affect the quality of your sleep by making you more restless? The same goes for eating heavy or spicy foods (such as *boeuf bourguignon* or *escargots*!), not to mention alcohol! Getting a good quality sleep means being light on our digestive system.

**MY TIP**

Do what the French usually do: have a proper lunch. This way, you will not feel the need to have a heavy meal at night. The added bonus to eating a more substantial lunch is having fewer cravings for sweets or fatty snacks in the afternoon!

## Transform your bedroom into a resting cocoon

If you want to get a good night's sleep, you should first check that your bedroom is really conducive to relaxation. Are you letting some fresh air in by opening the window every day? Is your mattress comfortable? Is your room warm enough or cool enough for you? And what about brightness and noise levels? These are important points to consider too as reducing sensory stimulation from light and sound can help us 'turn off' more easily.

**MY TIPS**

Wear an eye mask to block light if your bedroom is not dark enough. Wear some earplugs if you live in a noisy area or if your partner snores!

## Explore the wonderful benefits of aromatherapy

Aromatherapy can be very powerful: it can not only be used to treat physical ailments, it can also alter the way we feel by working on our brain via our sense of smell. Essential oils from botanicals can either have a stimulating or relaxing effect on our mind. So, why not use them to our advantage?

**MY TIPS**

Place a few drops of lavender or mandarin essential oils (or both) on a tissue and put it close to your pillow. Thanks to their calming effect on the mind, these essential oils promote relaxation (you can use these at any time of the day if you are feeling stressed: keep the scented tissue with you and inhale when needed). **Warning:** make sure that your oils are clearly labelled '100% pure essential oil' as you do not want to be breathing some ineffective or harmful synthetic fragrance.

# Living the 'skin-friendly' lifestyle means minimising your exposure to free radicals

An unhealthy lifestyle creates oxidative stress in our skin due to the action of free radicals. As we know, free radicals are harmful, and although our bodies have built-in mechanisms to fight and neutralise them, these defence mechanisms have limited powers. The best way to avoid skin damage and ageing caused by free radicals is to limit our exposure to them by altering our lifestyle.

## My suggestions for reducing your exposure to free radicals

### Limit your sun exposure

Exposure to UV rays causes free radical damage to our skin cells, and this precipitates the ageing process. However, a lot of people still spend too much time under the sun because they are afraid of being vitamin D deficient. The exact exposure time that we need to get sufficient levels of vitamin D can be difficult to establish as it can greatly vary depending on many factors including the colour of our skin, the country we live in, the season and the time of day. Having said that, this required exposure time is usually measured in minutes, not hours!

> **MY TIP**
>
> Are you concerned about your levels of vitamin D? If you think that you could be deficient, why not talk to your doctor about it. He/she will be able to give you more-specific information about your requirements and even organise a blood test to check your levels.

## Do not go to the solarium

Exposing our skin to the UV radiation from tanning beds is NOT less damaging or safer than prolonged and unprotected exposure to natural sunlight. As they mainly use deeply penetrating UVA rays, tanning beds can cause serious cellular damage and skin ageing, not to mention a drastic increase in your chance of developing skin cancer.

In my view, tanning beds SHOULD NOT exist. I am very pleased that, in Australia, some states have banned solariums. Hopefully, the rest of the world will follow.

**MY TIP**

If you really want to look tanned, use a self-tanning product.

## Limit your exposure to pollution

By now, we are all aware of the devastating effects that tobacco has on our health, and how smoking can speed up the ageing process of our skin by starving it of oxygen and nutrients. But one does not need to be a smoker to be exposed to the negative impact of air pollutants.

**MY TIP**

If you live in an urban environment, take regular trips and escape to the country. Your skin needs regular doses of fresh, clean air, and your soul some space and quietness!

# Living the 'skin-friendly' lifestyle means following a 'skin-friendly' diet

Feeding our skin from the inside is as important as caring for it on the outside. Indeed, what we ingest (or do not ingest) has an effect on the workings of our body and all its organs, including our skin. We kind of know this, having all experienced extra vitality when we follow a nutrient-rich diet and, conversely, feeling and looking rather under the weather when we have indulged in unhealthy foods for too long. So there is no point investing in good skincare products if we do not also take care of our skin's nutritional requirements!

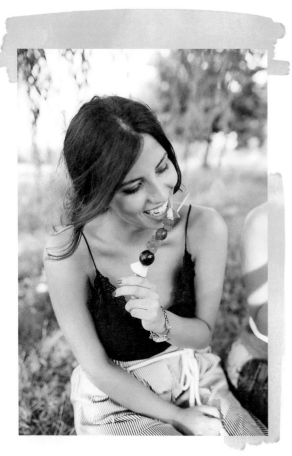

## My top 7 dietary guidelines to supercharge your skin

### *1. Eat a balanced diet*

Our skin thrives when fed a wide variety of fresh foods from each group – carbohydrates, proteins and fats (together with vitamins and minerals) – as our body needs these nutrients to function well and repair itself. Following strict and restrictive diets is not a good idea if you want your skin to glow (except, of course, for medical reasons).

> **MY TIPS**
>
> Shop at your local market rather than the supermarket: you will get fresh produce that is in season, meaning it is much more nutrient-rich and tasty.
>
> Cook your meals from scratch; it is much healthier than eating food that comes out of a packet. Share your culinary creations with your loved ones: this is not only healthier for your body, it is also wonderful for your soul!
>
> Do what French women do: eat a little of everything rather than a lot of a few things.
>
> Do not classify food as 'good' or 'bad': have it all in moderation. This is *très français!*

## 2. Eat enough protein

It is easy for women not to consume enough protein, especially if you are not into devouring juicy steaks or fish on a regular basis. This is something that we should keep in mind, as consuming an adequate amount of protein is crucial to maintaining skin firmness and boosting skin repair and health. Protein-rich foods do not only include meat, poultry and fish. Eggs, dairy products, legumes, avocados, nuts, sesame seeds, sunflower seeds and wheat germ all make the list too.

**ADDITIONAL RESOURCE**

For more nutritional information on all your dietary needs including proteins, visit the Australian Better Health Channel website at www.betterhealth.vic.gov.au. This is a fantastic resource from the State Government of Victoria, which covers healthy living in general (and even mental health). All useful to our skin! And guess what: it is also available as a free mobile phone app. *Parfait!*

## 3. Eat the good fats

We need essential fatty acids (EFAs), also known as omega-6s and omega-3s, in our diets as our bodies cannot synthesise them. These contribute to protecting our skin against premature ageing since they are involved in a number of important bodily roles including the fight against inflammation. They are also required to maintain the resilience of our cells.

Food sources of omega-3s include flaxseed oil, almonds, sesame seeds, avocado, kale, wheat germ oil, salmon, tuna and sardines. And you can find omega-6s in flaxseed oil, grapeseed oil, pumpkin seeds, sunflower seeds, olive oil, borage oil and evening primrose oil, among others.

**ADDITIONAL RESOURCE**

For more nutritional information on all your dietary needs including essential fatty acids, visit the Australian Better Health Channel website at www.betterhealth.vic.gov.au.

## 4. Eat more fruits and vegetables

Fruits and vegetables were a hot topic at the Anti-Ageing Skincare Conference that I attended in London in 2014. As I always encourage my own clients to eat more plant-based foods to support their skin, it was very pleasing to listen to some of the world's top skin scientists also lauding the anti-ageing effect of fruit and vegetables! Plant-based foods contain thousands and thousands of phytonutrients, all working in synergy to boost our health and help us combat the negative action of free radicals on our body. This is why they make such a great skin food.

### MY TIPS

A good way to ensure a broad intake of phytonutrients is to eat a wide variety of seasonal fruits and vegetables from the full 'rainbow' of colours of the plant world, and also to keep on changing your selection every day.

Do not forget your berries! They are such delicious and powerful antioxidants!

I personally take a natural fruit and vegetable supplement called Juice Plus to make sure that I get a wider range of fruits and vegetables in my daily diet (on top of eating quite a lot of them!). The scientific research done on this particular product shows that it has positive effects on the skin: a 39 per cent increase in the skin's microcirculation after three months, together with a 9 per cent increase in skin hydration, a 6 per cent increase in skin thickness and a 16 per cent increase in skin density. **Warning:** you should always consult your doctor before taking any dietary supplement.

(S. De Spirt, H. Sies, H. Tronnier & U. Heinrich, 'An encapsulated fruit and vegetable juice concentrate increases skin microcirculation in healthy women', Skin Pharmacology and Physiology, 2012;25(1):2-8 doi:10.1159/000330521)

## 5. Eat more raw food

The raw food movement is currently taking the world by storm. It consists of eating foods, usually plant-based, as close to their raw state as possible, which means either uncooked, or heated (or dehydrated) at no more than 118 degrees Celsius. The principle behind this eating philosophy is to keep intact all the vitamins, minerals and digestive enzymes present in the food we eat rather than having them destroyed by cooking.

**Please note:** I am not advocating that you should adhere to any extreme raw food diet, I just believe that it makes sense to include some raw food in our daily diet so as to get the most nutrition out of our food.

> **MY TIPS**

Experience the incredible power of raw, living ingredients by eating salads at every meal. Be creative and prepare your own French *salade de crudités*: a selection of raw vegetables on a bed of lettuce. It could be a mix of shredded beetroot and carrot, thin slices of tomato and cucumber, half a diced avocado, some artichoke, a little sweet corn, some fresh parsley and a few olives, or whatever else is in season. The secret is in the French dressing: in a jar, place 2 tablespoons of extra-virgin olive oil for every tablespoon of apple cider vinegar. Add some salt and pepper as well as Dijon mustard (careful, it is hot!). Close the lid, shake well and pour over your salad. *Voilà!*

If you find it hard to eat raw vegetables, drink them! For green smoothie recipes and other great resources, it is well worth visiting www.rawfamily.com

If you feel like dessert, choose raw desserts over the traditional sugar- and butter-laden baked options. For scrumptious raw dessert recipes (and many other dishes), check out the website of British raw chef Russell James: www.therawchef.com

You should also find great sweets at any of the raw food cafés and restaurants that are popping up everywhere. For a comprehensive list of Australian raw food cafés and restaurants, check out www.therawfoodmum.com/raw-cafes-and-restaurants-in-australia-new-zealand/

## 6. Eat less sugar

Sadly for the sweet-tooth crowd out there (including *moi!*), eating too much sugar is bad for our health as it encourages inflammation in the body. At a skin level, indulging in sugar causes our dermal collagen to undergo cross-linking (this happens when chemical attachments form between sugar and our collagen fibres), resulting in the formation of wrinkles. So, if you are serious about slowing down skin ageing, keep your sugar consumption to a minimum.

**MY TIPS**

An easy way to reduce your sugar intake is to stop drinking it. *Au revoir* sugary soft drinks, sweet alcoholic beverages and sweetened coffee!

Watch out for the hidden sugar added to a lot of processed foods, and remember that a simple home-cooked meal made from fresh and whole ingredients is always best.

*Traditionally, the French only eat cake on Sunday. Midmorning, they go to their favourite pâtisserie (cake shop) and patiently wait their turn to buy a selection of desserts. Baba au rhum, tarte au chocolat, clafouti aux cerises or éclair au café? So many to choose from . . . Do what the French do: have some dessert as a weekly treat and enjoy it thoroughly without feeling guilty. No need to become obsessive about things!*

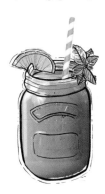

## 7. Drink more water

As our bodies contain a high proportion of water, good hydration promotes a properly functioning organism and vibrant skin. Health experts usually recommend that one should drink an average of 1.5 to 2 litres of fluids a day. Of course, water is the best source of hydration, followed by herbal teas, fresh vegetable juices, and also fruit juices (but in moderation because of their high sugar content).

### MY TIPS

It is best to avoid caffeine-based drinks such as coffee, tea and cola, as well as alcoholic beverages, as they all dehydrate the body. If you do consume these drinks, have an extra glass of water to compensate for this fluid loss.

This is a tip borrowed from my dear friend Freddy: to ensure that you drink enough fluids throughout the day, get into the habit of having a big glass of water every hour, on the hour.

*Eat* your water by munching on some extra fruits and vegetables. Plant foods have a high water content and, as we know, so many skin-friendly nutrients. *Pommes, framboises, carottes, tomates, aubergines . . . c'est trop bon!*

*Think of fruits and vegetables as hydrating and anti-ageing agents for your skin.*

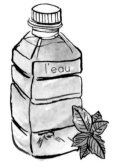

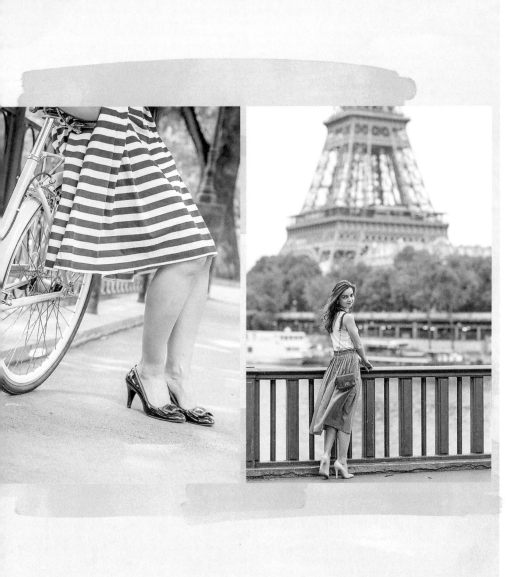

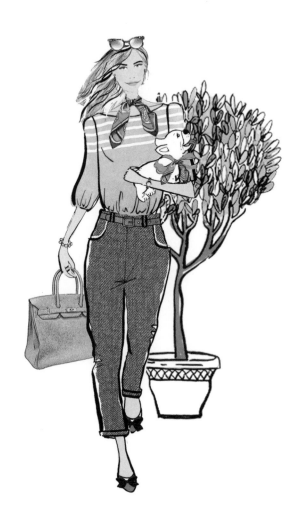

# CHAPTER 8

# HEALING
# YOUR SKIN

# Energetic healing

While the 'physical' factors for helping you achieve beautiful skin discussed in this book so far – skincare rituals, diet, sun protection – are all crucial to the health and appearance of your complexion, the 'non-physical' field also has the potential to have a huge impact on the state of your skin. This is the field of energetic healing. I am aware that a lot of people do not give much credence to such disciplines, but I have seen and learnt enough to be 100 per cent convinced.

## My experience with healing

I have had my own unequivocal healing experience via the hands of a healer. I was in my mid-twenties, living in Paris and slowly recovering from an operation that had left my left foot and leg feeling numb and ankylosed. In fact, I was so worried about it that I was ready to try anything to get better. On the advice of a colleague I decided to book a session with his healer, who had her practice next to Boulevard Montparnasse in the 14th arrondissement.

It was a short appointment: as soon as I arrived, Brigitte invited me to lie face-up and fully clothed on a massage bed. She then placed her hands over my head and proceeded to slowly move them all the way down my body to eventually reach my feet. After a few minutes, I felt what I would describe as a warm ball of energy shooting up my leg, as if something had been unblocked. It was a powerful sensation: it felt as if my circulation had suddenly been restored to its full capacity. I could feel my foot again! What a relief! I left feeling slightly overwhelmed by the intensity of what had just taken place and with a distinct improvement in my walk.

I will never forget this experience. This was the beginning of my journey into the realm of energy and healing. Today, I am a qualified reiki practitioner and I use healing energy during my facial treatments.

## Fire stoppers

During a recent visit to France, I watched one of my brother's DVDs, *Enquêtes Extraordinaires: Les Guérisseurs* by Thierry Machado. This documentary explored the healing world and the unexplained use of energy in the treatment of various physical diseases and ailments including those relating to the skin. Before watching it, I had never heard of 'fire stoppers'. These skin healers are so called because they are able to help heal skin burns caused by such things as fire, sunburn, hot water, radiotherapy or acid. They are able to 'stop the fire'. They are not only able to significantly relieve the deep pain associated with the most severe skin burns, but they can also greatly reduce scarring and accelerate the healing of the most serious cases of skin lesions. The documentary revealed that some French and Swiss hospitals implicitly recognise the favourable results of fire stoppers. In these hospitals, medical staff work hand in hand with skin healers to help relieve their patients' suffering and facilitate skin healing.

Having witnessed first-hand the devastating effects of skin burns on the life of burns victims, through my past volunteering with an Australian burns victims association, I felt compelled to find out more about these people and their reputed ability to facilitate skin healing through faith and spirituality. I was able to connect with two French fire stoppers online, Geneviève and Ricardo, who confirmed their respective skin healing powers. I was also able to interview Dr Clare Munday (better know as Dr Guillemin), who witnessed fire stoppers at work in the Clinique de La Source in Lausanne, Switzerland, while she was medical director of radio-oncology services there.

Dr Munday, a British medical practitioner, is a specialist in the field of integrative oncology. Her treatment methodology combines a sound scientific knowledge and medical experience with a more holistic approach to healing. While Dr Munday believes that the role of fire stoppers in the treatment of severe skin burns should not replace mainstream medical care, she can definitively attest to its pain relief benefits, saying: 'Whether or not this is a placebo effect or a spiritual effect, it does not really matter as the effect is very real.'

Dr Munday goes on to talk more broadly about the importance of our belief systems in relation to our own health and healing. 'Symptoms of ill-health are often manifestations of a complex internal terrain where biology interrelates with psychology, emotions, the physical as well as our beliefs,' she says. For her, everyone can be a catalyst to their own recovery as long as one believes in their capacity for healing. And, as a doctor, she sees herself as a co-creator of her patients' healing as long as they have faith in the treatment process. I feel the same about about skin health and my work as a facialist. This holistic connection between our physical skin's health and our state of mind is being investigated in the emerging field of 'psychodermatology'.

I witness first-hand this mind–skin interaction every day. For instance, it is quite common for skin disorders such as acne, dermatitis or rosacea to get worse during times of high emotional stress. I am not saying that emotions alone are the cause of such skin ailments, but they certainly can play a significant role in their development or their worsening. Emotions can physically affect the condition of our skin, and vice versa. You simply cannot separate the mind from the skin and the skin from the mind.

*If you want to positively transform your skin, the starting point must always be one of self-love and self-acceptance.*

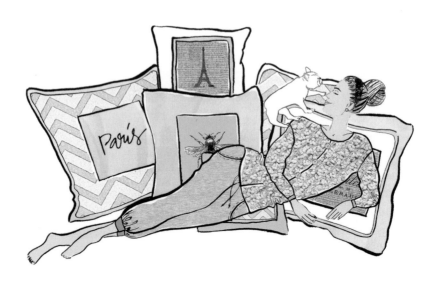

# Healing our skin with our thoughts

I am absolutely convinced that an accepting and loving state of mind is essential to any successful skincare approach. When a new client expresses their concerns and dislikes about the way their skin looks, I always encourage them to have a 'mind shift' about their skin. By 'mind shift', I mean starting to make friends with their skin right now, regardless of its current condition.

Most of us have been so hard on ourselves for so long that we have become accustomed to our daily dose of self-criticism about the way we look. It is so easy to tell ourselves: 'I will start liking myself when my skin gets clear of acne,' or 'If only I did not look so old . . .' Is it any wonder we forget how fundamentally linked to our psyche and emotions our skin truly is?

But, given the strong connection that exists between our mind and our skin, our thoughts trigger emotions which have an effect on our physiology, in a positive or negative way. I would even go further and suggest that the way we think about our skin, together with our skincare and lifestyle choices, influences how our skin looks, ages and regenerates. When we stop seeing our skin as imperfect, but rather start looking at it in a more positive and caring way, we trigger an inner feeling of self-love and healing that radiates beyond our skin.

*Loving is healing.*
*Healing is loving.*
*Simple.*

But, if we constantly criticise our skin by focusing on its every perceived flaw or if we let ourselves become overwhelmed by the fear of ageing, we create an unhealthy emotional environment that destabilises our entire system and adversely affects our skin.

So, why not begin to treat ourselves with more love and compassion by utilising the healing power of our thoughts?

## Creative visualisation

Here is my creative visualisation technique to 'tune' your thoughts and bring healing to your skin:

1.  **Find a quiet place.** It could be in your own home, in a park, at the beach . . . anywhere you like, where you can have some privacy. Find a comfortable spot and ease yourself into a relaxing position (personally, I find lying down best).

2.  **Close your eyes and take three long, deep breaths.** As you breathe in through your nose, your belly should expand as it takes the air in. As you breathe out through your mouth, it should flatten to its original state. Do not force your breathing; just go with the flow. By your third breath, you should find your breathing has become naturally deeper and you should be much more relaxed.

3.  **Focus your mind on your 'third eye'.** The 'third eye' is located between your eyes, in the centre of your forehead. It is said to be linked to deep thinking, self-imagery and intuition. Now, keep your attention clearly directed to this point.

4.  **Start visualising a beam of light coming out of your third eye.** You might 'see' white light or you might see colours. It does not matter what image you perceive. This experience varies from one person to the next.

5.  **Keep visualising the beam of light and begin to feel its energy.** As you focus on the light beam, you may sense some associated heat or vibrations. You may also experience a deep feeling of love or compassion. Again, this is a personal journey that is unique to you. Whatever form this beam of light has, it is the right one for you. Keep visualising and feeling the light energy amplify.

6.  **Start expanding the flow of light to your entire face.** As you mentally direct the flow of light from your third eye to your whole face, feel its healing energy envelop the skin of your forehead, your nose, your cheeks, your ears, your mouth, your chin and around your jawline. Focus your intention on the deep healing that is taking place. Feel the light penetrate your skin, down to the core of your skin, bathing all your skin cells and the spaces between them.

7.  **Continue by expanding the flow of light to your entire body.** Slowly now

infuse your whole body with this loving and healing light. Let it expand and cover your neck, your shoulders, your arms down to the tips of your fingers, your chest, your abdomen, your legs, right down to the tips of your toes. Visualise and feel the light wrapping your entire body with deep love and a feeling of peace.

8. **Stay still for a few minutes and enjoy this feeling of inner peace.** All is well in your world. All is the way it is meant to be right now. Feel the sensation of deep love and compassion. You are unique. You are perfect the way you are. It is time to let the light shine throughout your entire life. It is time to be happy, exactly the way you are, right now.

9. **Take three long, deep breaths and start becoming aware of your external environment.** Stretch your body and slowly open your eyes. Observe how peaceful and light you are feeling. You are alive and well. You are love. You are light.

10. **Repeat this visualisation as often as you like.** The more you practise this technique, the easier it will become to visualise the light and immerse yourself in it.

**Note:** Do this exercise every time your skin is in need of healing (for instance, if you are experiencing some acne, eczema or rosacea flare-ups), when you look and feel fatigued or even when you feel a wave of self-doubt or self-criticism.

If you are unable to go through this entire visualisation exercise (you may be at work or may not be able to physically retreat to a private place), you can always mentally tap into this feeling of deep love and inner peace by focusing on your third eye and visualising being surrounded by its healing light. You can do this wherever you are, whatever your environment.

# Healing our skin with our touch

Our hands can also be the vehicles for an endless source of healing energy. The need to heal or be healed through touch is innate in us humans. To comprehend this, you only need to watch a mother instinctively applying her hand onto the knee of her child who has just fallen and hurt himself; or observe yourself placing your hand onto the shoulder of a friend needing reassurance or comfort. We can all use a simple facial massage to tap into the healing benefits of touch. Massage is an effective way to assist our skin's self-regeneration process (it encourages the circulation of blood and lymph, helping bring nutrition to our skin cells and assisting the skin in its detoxification). It encourages the release of emotional stress that can detrimentally affect our facial tissues, and it can also be a loving expression of self-care.

## Self-healing facial massage for skin rejuvenation

This self-massage should always be performed on clean skin and with clean hands, so as not to massage in any dirt or grime. I also recommend that you moisturise your skin prior to getting started. A little moisturiser (or even a thin layer of a hydrating mask) will give your skin the right conditioning to allow for enough 'glide' without feeling too greasy. It can also help if you use a mirror until you get accustomed to this facial routine.

1. **Find a comfortable position.** It could be standing up or sitting down; whatever you prefer, as long as you are feeling relaxed.
2. **Start by quickly rubbing your hands together for about ten seconds.** This is to generate some heat between your hands.
3. **Close your eyes and cover your face with both hands.** Your hands should be lightly resting on each side of your face, fingers facing up towards your hairline and elbows resting on your chest. For a minute or so, with your hands still, focus on the heat emanating from your hands. Mentally observe the flow of energy travelling through your hands onto your skin.
4. **Perform light tapping movements all over your face.** Tapping with each finger individually like a ripple, repeat this up and down your entire face six times. It should feel like little drops of rain falling on your face.

5. **Perform light spiral movements on your forehead.** Starting in the middle of your forehead, perform slow spirals with your fingertips from the midline of the forehead towards your temples. Go back and forth over the entire forehead six times.

6. **Continue with pressure points over the eye area.** Starting under the eyes, with your fingertips resting on your orbital bones (around the eye socket), press lightly on a sequence of points, as you move your fingertips from the inner to the outer corner of your eyes. Repeat six times.

7. **Moving both hands at the same time, perform rolling movements on your cheeks.** With the fingers of each hand pressed together and fingertips pointing upwards, rest your palms on your cheeks, the little fingers touching the sides of your nose. Gently roll your hands while moving them towards your ears and then back towards your nose. Repeat six times.

8. **Repeat step 4.** Perform light tapping movements all over your face.

9. **Perform stroking movements all over your face.** With the pads of your fingers, gently stroke your skin as if you were spreading a moisturiser over your face. Start with your forehead, going upwards from your eyebrows to your hairline and down towards your temples, sweep under the eyes towards your temples. Sweep over your cheeks and your chin. Finish with a downward stroking movement over your neck and décolletage. Repeat this sequence three times.

10. **Repeat steps 2 and 3.** Focus on directing your energy to each and every one of your skin cells, washing away all the tensions, all the stress and all the pressures of everyday life.

11. **Repeat weekly or more often if you feel any facial tension developing.**

# The secret to having skin that you love

Paradoxically, and because of the mind–skin link, the secret to having skin that we love must begin with accepting and respecting what we are and how we look, right now, regardless of the fact that there may be some aspects of our complexion that we might like to work on. We must start by loving our skin right now, no matter its current condition! Easier said than done?

There are many tips and tools to help with self-acceptance. I particularly find the following to be very effective:

## 1. Stop comparing yourself with others

Comparing our physical appearance with others' is counterproductive. In fact, it can easily make us feel insecure and inadequate (of course there will always be someone around who is younger and prettier, with clearer skin!). Instead, let's acknowledge and celebrate the fact that we are all unique and that we have the skin that we are meant to have right now.

> **MY TIP**
>
> I particularly like this quote by the late American actor Jack Lord, which I find inspirational: 'What you have, what you are – your looks, your personality, your way of thinking – is unique. No one in the world is like you. So capitalize on it.'

## 2. Be realistic about your expectations

There is no such thing as 'flawless' skin: this is an absolute myth that is sadly being perpetuated by the media and the beauty industry. Always remember that fashion magazines photoshop their pictures to erase all skin imperfections and wrinkles. Even the most beautiful-looking models do not have perfect skin. So let's stop buying into this lie and watch our sense of inner power grow!

> **MY TIP**
>
> Change your mindset around perfection. Nothing about life, ourselves or the way we look is 100 per cent perfect. It is a fact! Wanting to be and look perfect is fighting a losing battle. We are human and imperfection is part of the human experience.

### 3. Be proactive and take control

If you truly believe that your skin could look better than it does at the moment, it is time to be brutally honest with yourself: are you doing everything in your power to have your skin looking its best? Always remember that you do have the power to positively influence the way your skin behaves and looks.

**MY TIP**

Know that, being a living organ, your skin is in a constant state of change. This means that it can always improve. No need to feel powerless and frustrated in regards to your skin!

### 4. Exercise 'ESC'

I am a big fan of 'extreme self-care', a great term that I first heard from my American friend Cindy. Taking time out to give back and nurture yourself is not selfish but is truly essential to your sense of happiness and wellbeing. In spite of your numerous life commitments, make time for YOU on a regular basis (even if it is only 30 minutes a week). Spend this time doing something that you love, something that makes you feel good (walking in the park, reading a book, having a bath, putting a facial mask on, eating your favourite treat . . . ).

**MY TIP**

Diarise that 'ESC' time. Make this appointment with yourself absolutely non-negotiable, and as crucial as any other important meetings that you might have with others.

### 5. Reflect on your life

Why is it that we can like our physical features one particular day and feel the exact opposite about ourselves the next? Loving or resenting the way we look is not always linked to our appearance itself. In fact, it is often symptomatic of other things that are going on in our lives: it is easier to beat ourselves up about the way we look rather than dealing with the real reasons why we feel lousy. Looking deeper within might feel a little uncomfortable at first, and our initial reaction might be to brush things off. That is totally fine. But be persistent: it is only by becoming aware of unresolved issues in our life that we can start acting on them. And this always leads to a reinforced feeling of (much needed) self-love.

> **MY TIP**

Stop for a moment, take a deep breath and feel what is going on within you. Ask yourself: 'Which emotions am I experiencing? Is it anger, fear, guilt or sadness? Where is this coming from? What is triggering these feelings?' Every time you get an answer, push a little further by questioning that answer, asking yourself, 'Why?' Keep asking 'Why?' and you will soon get to the core of the real issue. It is so much easier to change the things that do not serve us when we know what they actually are!

## 6. Practise daily affirmations

We can all be so self-critical; sometimes without even realising it. A powerful self-acceptance tool is the regular use of positive affirmations as a way to counteract the negative inner chatter that can affect our self-image.

> **MY TIP**

Every day, stand in front of your mirror, close your eyes for a few seconds, take several deep breaths, open your eyes, look at yourself clearly and, with compassion, tell yourself out loud several times: '*I deeply and completely love and accept myself.*'

## 7. Read the wise words of your favourite self-help writer

Since we all need regular support and encouragement to get to our own place of self-love, reading self-help books and blogs can be very constructive. Indeed, considering others' reflections on life can help us find our own answers quicker. And it can also be an external source of comfort knowing that we all share similar life struggles, hopes and dreams.

As mentioned earlier, I get a lot out of reading the blog of Leo Babauta. This is an extract from Leo's blog entry titled 'Unconditional Acceptance of Yourself' (posted on 26 January 2015). Be sure to go to his site and read the full post (see link below). *Merci*, Leo! *'Acceptance isn't stagnation – you will change no matter what. You can't avoid changing. The question is whether that change comes from a place of acceptance and love, or a place of self-dislike and dissatisfaction. I vote for unconditional love.'* (www.zenhabits.net/unconditional)

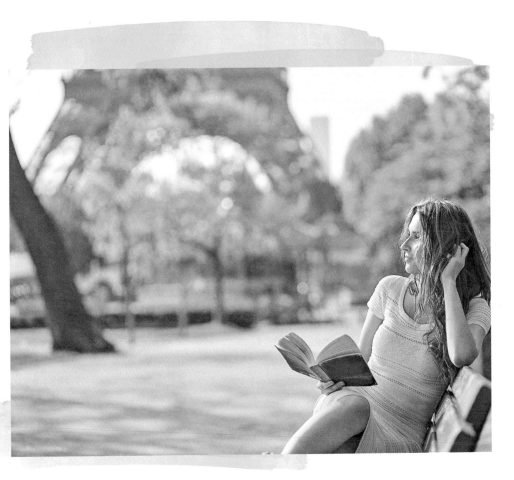

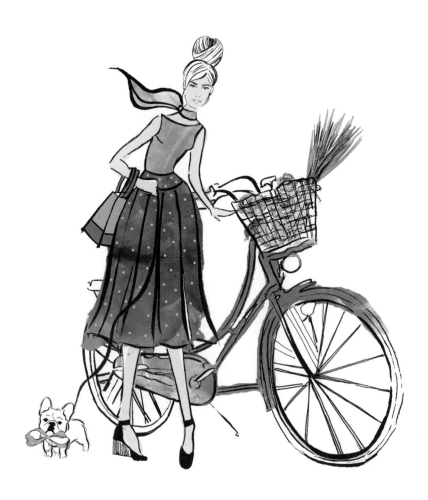

# CONCLUSION
## VOILÀ

# Action plan for happy skin

## I shall . . . practise self-love
- read 'Manifesto for happy skin' every day
- choose to see the best in myself and others
- always keep in mind that perfection is a myth
- reflect on the fact that I am TRULY special (there is only one of ME)

## I shall . . . acknowledge my own needs
- take the time to find out what I need to feel happy and balanced
- say 'no' to people without feeling guilty or wanting to justify myself
- only say 'yes' to people when I really mean it
- say 'yes' to nurturing myself more often

## I shall . . . relax and rest
- not worry about things that may never happen
- spend some time alone or meditate daily, even if only briefly
- switch off my mobile phone, computer and television for at least one hour a day
- get some beauty sleep (aim to go to bed before 10 p.m.)

## I shall . . . nurture my skin every day
- perform my skincare rituals every morning and every night, no matter what!

## I shall . . . pamper my skin at any opportunity
- perform a mini home facial once a week (cleanse, exfoliate, mask & moisturise)
- practise self-healing techniques on my skin
- have a professional facial with a reputable facialist
- treat myself to a massage or a spa treatment

## I shall . . . avoid damaging my skin

- say '*non, merci*' to facial cleansing brushes, pads and loofahs
- never go to solariums
- not over-exfoliate my skin
- not use harsh products on my skin
- treat my skin gently (not be rough!)

## I shall . . . be sun smart

- avoid sun exposure when the UV index is 3 or above
- wear high SPF (30+ or higher) broad spectrum sunscreen when the UV index is 3 or above
- cover my skin with light-coloured clothing when the UV index is 3 or above
- wear high-quality sunglasses when the UV index is 3 or above
- wear a wide-brimmed hat when the UV index is 3 or above

## I shall . . . boost my skin from the inside out

- have a green smoothie every day
- eat at least five serves of vegetables and two serves of fruit each day
- eat more raw foods
- eat more skin-friendly foods such as salmon or tuna
- take a skin-boosting supplement

## I shall . . . tune up my lifestyle habits constantly

- not smoke, and get plenty of fresh air
- drink more water, herbal teas or vegetable juices
- have at least three alcohol-free days a week
- reduce or eliminate processed foods and added sugar from my diet
- walk more

## And finally, I shall . . . add a splash of colour to my life

- wear bright-coloured clothes
- experiment with make-up and have fun with it
- wear bright lipstick
- choose to see the bright and colourful side of life
- smile and laugh every day

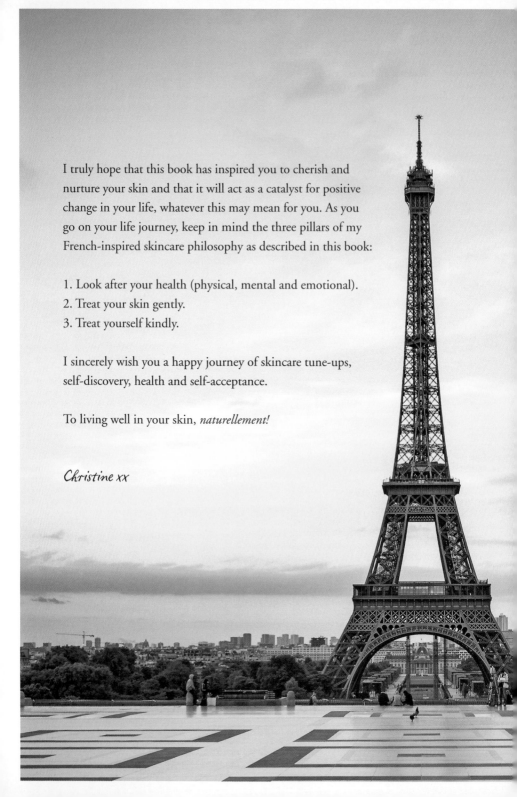

I truly hope that this book has inspired you to cherish and nurture your skin and that it will act as a catalyst for positive change in your life, whatever this may mean for you. As you go on your life journey, keep in mind the three pillars of my French-inspired skincare philosophy as described in this book:

1. Look after your health (physical, mental and emotional).
2. Treat your skin gently.
3. Treat yourself kindly.

I sincerely wish you a happy journey of skincare tune-ups, self-discovery, health and self-acceptance.

To living well in your skin, *naturellement!*

*Christine xx*

# *Merci*

This book would not have been created without the valued support of the following people.

**Penguin Books Australia team**
An immeasurable thank you for helping me make this book – and my dream – a reality. Un grand merci à vous, Arwen Summers, Cate Blake and Grace West.

**Alexia Pitsinis, illustrator** (www.alexiapetsinis.com)
You are such a joy to work with and talented far beyond your years. Thank you for giving life to our beloved 'Charlotte' and 'J.J.' and staying true to my illustrative vision.

**Victoria Martin, make-up artist** (www.victoriamartin.co.uk)
Your expert contribution to this book is tremendously appreciated. Thank you for divulging your insider make-up secrets and sharing how to use colour to our beautiful advantage.

**Dr Clare Munday** (better known as Dr Clare Guillemin), holistic medical practitioner (www.drclaremunday.ch, www.vielavie.ch, www.alpalamas.ch)
Thank you for sharing your positive views on health and healing as well as advocating a medical approach that allows patients to actively participate in their recovery.

**My clients – past and present**
I am sincerely grateful to every single one of you for entrusting me with your skin. In essence, you are all contributors to this book because you've helped shape and refine my skincare philosophy.

**Lina, my treasured friend and colleague for more than twenty years**
Thank you for your dear friendship and being a valuable sounding-board for the content of this book.

**Christophe, my life partner**
Words are not enough to express my thanks for your constant support and for enriching my life.

**Marcel, Juliette and Lily – my furry kids**
Thank you for being such loyal writing companions.

# Product list

Following is a list of the skincare products and cosmetics mentioned in this book.

It is important to note that I have not been paid to endorse any of the products recommended in this book. I have purely suggested particular items that I genuinely like and seen have a positive effect on my clients' skin as well as my own complexion.

I have classified products into various age categories as a general guide – this means you could still choose products from other age brackets, if you feel that they relate to you and will benefit your skin. In any case, always make sure to consider your skin type and condition before your age.

Of course, there are many other great skincare choices on the market, so I would encourage you to give other products a try too. Remember, however, when shopping for new skincare: always focus on ingredients and their intended action on skin, not the packaging!

Finally, please make sure that you refer to the manufacturer's instructions before using any new skincare product and discontinue use if irritation occurs.

(L) indicates a 'luxe' product – over $100.

**Please note:** The recommendations made in this book are provided as general advice and based on my extensive skincare experience and best intentions – that is, optimising the condition of your skin. For a more tailored skin analysis and treatment plan (that takes into account your specific circumstances), please consult a skincare specialist.

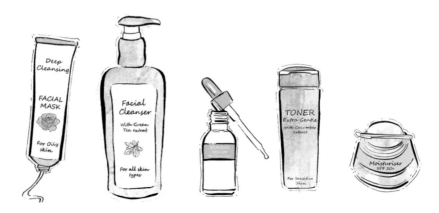

## LATE TEENS AND TWENTIES – SKINCARE PRODUCTS

### CLEANSERS
- Skin Juice Eden Smoothing Cleansing Cream (normal to oily skin)
- Image Skincare Ormedic Balancing Facial Cleanser (all skin types)

### TONERS
- Institut Esthederm Osmoclean Alcohol Free Calming Lotion (sensitive or sensitised skin)
- Skin Juice Multi Juice Balancing Tonic (oily, combination or blemish-prone skin)

### EYE CARE
- Uskincare Revital Eyes Eyelift Gel (all skin types)
- Clarins Eye Contour Balm (all skin types)

### MOISTURISERS
- Sukin Facial Moisturiser (all skin types)
- Skin Juice Citrus Oil Control Face Cream (oily, combination skin or blemish-prone skin)

### SERUMS
- Skin Juice Liquid Tri Active Clearing Serum (oily, combination skin or blemish-prone skin)
- Sircuit Skin Cosmeceuticals Fixzit Blemish Drying Serum (spot treatment)

### EXFOLIANTS
- Skin Juice Pulp Clarifying Cleansing Paste (oily, combination skin or blemish-prone skin)
- Uskincare Bamboo Polish (all skin types except sensitised skin)

### MASKS
- Palmer's Cocoa Butter Formula Purifying Enzyme Mask (oily, combination skin or blemish-prone skin)
- Antipodes Aura Manuka Honey Mask (dehydrated, blemish-prone skin)

## THIRTIES – SKINCARE PRODUCTS

### CLEANSERS
- Sircuit Skin Cosmeceuticals Supermild Sensitive Skin Cleansing Crème (all skin types)
- Institut Esthederm Osmoclean Pure Cleansing Foam (combination to oily skin)

### TONERS
- Sukin Hydrating Mist Toner (all skin types)
- Gernetic Fibro (all skin types except sensitised skin)

### EYE CARE
- Bliss Triple Oxygen Instant Energizing Eye Gel (all skin types)
- Antipodes Kiwi Seed Oil Eye Cream (all skin types)

### MOISTURISERS
- Indeed Laboratories Hydraluron Moisture Jelly (all skin types)
- Institut Esthederm Hydra System Aqua Diffusion Care Cream (all skin types)

### SERUMS
- Skin Juice Shine Resurfacing Serum (all skin types)
- Sircuit Skin Cosmeceuticals Sircuit Weapon 10% Vitamin C Therapy Serum (L) (all skin types)

### EXFOLIANTS
- Sircuit Skin Cosmeceuticals Sir Activ Zeolite Invigorating Scrub (all skin types except sensitised skin)
- Dermalogica Daily Microfoliant (all skin types)

### MASKS
- Bliss Triple Oxygen Instant Energizing Mask (all skin types except sensitive or sensitised skin)
- Image Skincare Vital C Hydrating Enzyme Masque (all skin types)

## FORTIES – SKINCARE PRODUCTS

CLEANSERS
- Institut Esthederm Osmoclean Hydra-Replenishing Cleansing Milk (dehydrated or normal to dry skin)
- Uskincare Nourish Milk Cleanser (dehydrated or normal to dry skin)

TONERS
- Institut Esthederm Cellular Water Spray (all skin types)
- Sircuit Skin Cosmeceuticals Molecular Mist (all skin types)

EYE CARE
- Epicure Cosmeceuticals Skin Firming Eye Serum (L) (all skin types)
- Sircuit Skin Cosmeceuticals White Out Daily Under Eye Care (L) (all skin types)

MOISTURISERS
- Auriège Paris Chrono-V Revitalizing Global Care (L) (mature skin)
- Embryolisse Lait-Crème Concentré (dry and dehydrated skin)

SERUMS
- Image Skincare Ageless Total Anti-Aging Serum (L) (ageing, sun damaged or blemish-prone skin)
- Image Skincare Ageless Total Pure Hyaluronic Filler (L) (dry or dehydrated skin)

EXFOLIANTS
- Phytomer Vegetal Exfoliant with Natural Enzymes (all skin types)
- Gernetic Ger Peel (L) (all skin types except sensitised skin)

MASKS
- Gernetic Hydra Ger (L) (all skin types except highly sensitive or sensitised skin)
- Sircuit Skin Cosmeceuticals Cool Lychee Wa Intensely Hydrating Mask (L) (all skin types)

## FIFTIES AND BEYOND – SKINCARE PRODUCTS

CLEANSERS
- Skin Juice Drench Dermal Repair Cleansing Oil (dry, dehydrated skin, combination skin)
- Sothys Beauty Garden Make-Up Removing Fluid (all skin types)

TONERS
- Uskincare Damask Rose Hydrosol (all skin types)
- Embryolisse Eau de Beauté Rosamélis (all skin types)

EYE CARE
- Phytomer Expertise Age Contour Intense Youth Eye Cream (L) (all skin types)
- Epicure Cosmeceuticals Anti-Ageing Eye Serum: Liquid Crystal (L) (all skin types)

MOISTURISERS
- Epicure Cosmeceuticals Intensive Care Hydrator (dry, dehydrated and mature skin)
- Gernetic Cytobi (L) (dry, mature, sensitive and sensitised skin)

SERUMS
- Uskincare Sensitive Rescue Serum (dehydrated, sensitive and sensitised skin)
- Sircuit Skin Cosmeceuticals Nineoneone Calming Serum (L) (sensitive or sensitised skin)

EXFOLIANTS
- Institut Esthederm Osmoclean Gentle Deep Pore Cleanser (all skin types)
- Indeed Laboratories Facial Powdered Exfoliator (all skin types)

MASKS
- Avène Soothing Moisture Mask (dry or sensitive skin)
- Skin Juice Vanilla + Honey Moisture Massage Mask (dry or sensitive skin)

## ALL AGES – SKINCARE PRODUCTS

### EYE MAKE-UP REMOVERS
- Clarins Instant Eye Make-up Remover (waterproof)
- The Body Shop Camomile Gentle Eye Make-up Remover (non-waterproof)

### MULTI-PURPOSE CLEANSER
- Embryolisse Lotion Micellaire (all skin types)

### HYDRATORS
- La Roche-Posay Thermal Water Spray (all skin types)
- Evian Brumisateur Facial Spray (all skin types)

### SUNSCREENS
- La Roche-Posay Anthelios XL SPF 50+ Extreme Fluid (all skin types including sensitive skin)
- La Roche-Posay Anthelios XL SPF 50+ Melt-In Cream (dry skin including sensitive skin)
- Sunsational Clear Sunscreen SPF 50+ (all skin types)

### MOISTURISING SUNSCREEN
- O Cosmedics Mineral Pro SPF 30+ (all skin types)

## ADDITIONAL PRODUCTS FOR:

### FINE LINES AND WRINKLES
- Sircuit Skin Cosmeceuticals Mocha Loca Chocolate Lactic Acid Peel (L)
- Image Skincare Ageless Total Repair Crème (L)
- Image Skincare Ageless Total Eye Lift Crème
- Image Skincare The Max Stem Cell Eye Crème
- Image Skincare Ageless Total Pure Hyaluronic Filler (L)
- Embryolisse Artist Secret Complexion Illuminating Veil BB Cream
- Auriège Paris Lift CC Cream

### OPEN PORES
- Image Skincare Ageless Total Anti-Aging Serum (L)
- Epicure Cosmeceuticals Enzyme Peel: Pumpkin (L)
- Dermalogica Daily Microfoliant
- Embryolisse Artist Secret Complexion Illuminating Veil BB Cream
- By Terry Hyaluronic Hydra-Primer Colorless Hydra-Filler

### UNDER-EYE DARK CIRCLES AND PUFFINESS
- Epicure Skin Firming Eye Serum (L)

### BLACKHEADS, WHITEHEADS AND MILIA
- Image Skincare Ageless Total Pure Hyaluronic Filler (L)
- Indeed Laboratories Hydraluron Moisture Jelly
- Phytomer Vegetal Exfoliant with Natural Enzymes
- Image Skincare Vital C Hydrating Enzyme Masque

### ACNE
- Image Skincare Ormedic Balancing Facial Cleanser
- Image Skincare Vital C Hydrating Anti-Aging Serum
- Sircuit Skin Cosmeceuticals Sircuit Agent (L)
- Mineralogie Make-Up

### SENSITIVE AND SENSITISED SKIN
- Institut Esthederm Osmoclean High Tolerance Make-up Remover – Waterproof Eyes and Lips
- Institut Esthederm Sensi System Calming Eye Contour Cream
- La Roche-Posay Toleriane range

### DARK PIGMENTATION MARKS
- Sircuit Skin Cosmeceuticals Brilliance Fading Serum
- Gernetic Skin Clair Concentrate (L)

- Gernetic Skin Clair Nutritive Cream (L)
- Sircuit Skin Cosmeceuticals Double
  Trouble 5% Lactic Pomegranate Acai Peel
  (L)

## MAKE-UP SOLUTIONS (CHAPTER 6)

### PRIMING
- Embryolisse Lait-Crème Concentré
- By Terry Hyaluronic Hydra-Primer
  Colorless Hydra-Filler
- Hourglass Veil Mineral Primer SPF 15
- Tom Ford Illuminating Primer

### CONCEALING BLEMISHES
- Clé de Peau Beauté Concealer (L)
- Vichy Dermablend

### CONCEALING DARK CIRCLES
- Bobbi Brown Corrector
- Bobbi Brown Creamy Concealer
- Ellis Faas Concealer

### DEALING WITH DROOPY EYELIDS
- Shu Uemura Eyelash Curler

### MINIMISING THE APPEARANCE OF WRINKLES
- By Terry Hyaluronic Hydra-Powder

## MAKE-UP ESSENTIALS (CHAPTER 6)

### LATE TEENS AND TWENTIES
- NARS Semi Matte Lipstick in 'Schiap'
- NARS Sheer Lipstick in 'Roman Holiday'
- MAC Face and Body Foundation
- Clé de Peau Beauté Concealer (L)

### THIRTIES
- Chanel Rouge Coco Shine lipstick in
  'Rebelle'
- Clarins Joli Rouge Lipstick in 'Clarins Red'
- MAC 'Ruby Woo' Lipstick
- Urban Decay Naked Eyeshadow Palette
- Bobbi Brown Corrector
- Bobbi Brown Creamy Concealer

### FORTIES
- Clarins Beauty Flash Balm
- Bobbi Brown Long-Wear Cream Shadow
  in 'Shore'
- Bobbi Brown Long-Wear Cream Shadow in
  'Velvet Plum'
- By Terry Crayon Khol Terrybly

### FIFTIES AND BEYOND
- Kevin Aucoin The Volume Mascara
- Lipstick Queen Invisible Lip Liner
- Anastasia Berverly Hills Brow Wiz

# Bibliography

Atkinson, Mark, Holistic Health Secrets for Women, London, Piatkus Books, 2009.

Babauta, Leo, Zen Habits is about finding simplicity in the daily chaos of our lives, www.zenhabits.net.

Begoun, Paula (author of *Don't Go to the Cosmetics Counter Without Me*), www.paulaschoice.com/expert-advice/skincare-advice.

Better Health Channel, Food and Nutrition, www.betterhealth.vic.gov.au/bhcv2/bhcarticles.nsf/pages/hl_foodnutrition?open.

Brennan, Barbara Ann, *Hands of Light: A Guide to Healing Through the Human Energy Field*, New York, Bantam Books, 1987.

Cancer Council Australia, Preventing Cancer, Sun Safety, www.cancer.org.au/preventing-cancer/sun-protection.

Dagognet, François, *La Peau Découverte*, Paris, Empecheurs De Penser En Rond, 1998.

Dick, Martin, *Origines et Pratiques des Anciens Tradithérapeutes*, Paris, Éditions du Dauphin, 2012.

Fisher, Karen, *The Healthy Skin Diet*, Wollombi, Exisle Publishing Limited, 2008.

James, Russell, The Raw Chef, www.therawchef.com.

Michalun, M Varinia and Joseph C DiNardo, *Milady's Skin Care and Cosmetic Ingredients Dictionary 4th Edition*, Clifton Park, Milady, 2014.

Mok, Kim, The Manifesto Manifesto, www.kimmok.com/the-manifesto-manifesto.

Lees, Mark, *Skin Care: Beyond the Basics*, Albany, Milady, 2001.

Lees, Mark, *The Skin Care Answer Book, First Edition*, Clifton Park, Milady, 2011.

Mélissopoulos, Alexandre and Christine Levacher, *La Peau*, Paris, Technique & Documentation, 1998.

Perricone, Nicholas, *The Wrinkle Cure*, New York, Warner Books, 2000.

Raw Family, The Green Smoothie Headquaters, www.rawfamily.com.

Smith, Pamela Wartian, *What You Must Know about Women's Hormones*, Garden City Park, Square One Publishers, 2010.

Stafford, Julie, *Juicing for Health*, Boston, Tuttle Publishing, Inc, 1998.

Sun Smart, UV & Sun Protection, www.sunsmart.com.au/uv-sun-protection.

Tortora, Gerard J. and Brian Derrickson, *Principles of Anatomy and Physiology*, Hoboken, John Wiley & Sons, Inc, 2009.

World Health Organization, UV Radiation, www.who.int/topics/ultraviolet_radiation/en.

# Stockist list

Anastasia Beverly Hills: Online: www.itbeginswithbrows.com.au.

Antipodes: Online and instore: www.priceline.com.au.

Auriège Paris: Online: www.thefrenchfacialist.com.

Avène: Online: www.priceline.com.au. Stockists: www.avene.com.au.

Bliss: Online and instore: www.priceline.com.au.

Bobbi Brown: Online and instore: www.bobbibrown.com.au.

By Terry: Online and instore: www.mecca.com.au.

Chanel: Online: www.davidjones.com.au. Stockists: www.chanel.com.

Clarins: Online and instore: www.myer.com.au.

Clé de Peau Beauté: Available online from www.skincaredirect.com.au.

Dermalogica: Online and instore: www.dermalogica.com.au.

Ellis Faas: Online and instore: www.mecca.com.au.

Embryolisse: Online: www.scottysmakeup.com.au. Stockists: www.embryolisse.com.au.

Epicure Cosmeceuticals: Sold exclusively by qualified skincare professionals.
    Online: www.beautyonburke.com.au. Stockists: call 03 9077 2135.

Evian: Online and instore www.chemistwarehouse.com.au.

Gernetic: Sold exclusively by qualified skincare professionals.
    Stockists: www.gernetic.com.au.

Hourglass: Online and instore: www.mecca.com.au.

Image Skincare: Sold exclusively by qualified skincare professionals.
    Stockists: www.imageskincare.com.au.

Indeed Laboratories: Online and instore: www.priceline.com.au.

Institut Esthederm: Online: www.derma-cosmetics.com.

Kevyn Aucoin: Online and instore: www.mecca.com.au.

La Roche-Posay: Online: www.priceline.com.au. Stockists: www.laroche-posay.com.au.

Lipstick Queen: Online and instore: www.mecca.com.au.

MAC: Online and instore www.maccosmetics.com.au.

Mineralogie Mineral Make-Up: Online and instore: www.mineralogie.com.au.

NARS: Online and instore: www.mecca.com.au.

O Cosmedics: Online and instore: www.inskincosmedics.com.au.

Palmer's Cocoa Butter Formula: Online: www.chemistwarehouse.com.au.
   Stockists: www.palmersaustralia.com.

Phytomer: Online: www.phytomer.com.au.

Shu Uemura: Online and instore: www.davidjones.com.au.

Sircuit Skin Cosmeceuticals: Sold exclusively by qualified skincare professionals.
   Stockists: call 1300 135 294.

Skin Juice: Online and instore: www.skinjuice.com.au.

Sothys: Sold exclusively by qualified skincare professionals. Stockists: www.sothys.com.au.

Sukin: Online and instore: www.sukinorganics.com.

Sunsational: Online: www.sunsationalbodycare.com.au. Stockists: call 02 9664 1412.

The Body Shop: Online and instore: www.thebodyshop.com.au.

Tom Ford: Online: www.davidjones.com.au. Stockists: www.tomford.com.

Urban Decay: Online and instore: www.mecca.com.au.

Uskincare: Online: www.uspa.com.au.

Vichy Dermablend: Online: www.escentual.com.

# Photography credits

Page ii: (left) by Eva Katalin Kondoros/Istock; (right) by malhrovitz/Istock; P4: author photograph by Simon Strong www.simonstrong.com; P13: (left) Vanni Bassetti/Getty Images; (right) Ekaterina Pokrovsky/Shutterstock; P19: Eva Katalin Kondoros/Istock; P20: Guille Faingold/Stocksy United; P24: (left) encrier/Istock; (right) Vanni Bassetti/Getty Images; P27: (left) Jovana Rikalo/Stocksy United; (right) Vanni Bassetti/Getty Images; P32: Sam Hurd/Stocksy United; P36: (left) Ekaterina Pokrovsky/Shutterstock; (right) Jovana Rikalo/Stocksy United; P39: Todor Tsvetkov/Istock; P52: (left) Matteo Colombo/Stocksy United; (right) encrier/Istock; P73: (left) Yuri Arcurs/Istock; (right) andresr/Istock; P80: SunKids/Shutterstock; P88: (left) GlobalStock/Istock; (right) gresei/Shutterstock; P97: (left) RossHelen/Shuttertsock; (right) Nicolesa/Shutterstock; P109: (left) gpointstudio/Istock; (right) Lars Zahner/Shutterstock; P114: Vladimir Volodin/Shutterstock; P117: (left and right) HconQ/Shutterstock; P129: fotostorm/Istock; P132: (left) Subbotina Anna/Shutterstock; (right) Shots Studio/Shutterstock; P141: Michela Ravasio/Stocksy United; P145: (left) alexalenin/Istock; (right) swissmediavision/Istock; P150: (left) AleksandarNakic/Istock; (right) kkgas/Stocksy United; P160: (left) Marko Milanovic/Stocksy United; (right) Alija/Istock; P178: Jovana Rikalo/Stocksy United; P185: (left) Pilin Petunyia/Istock; (right) Ekaterina Pokrovsky/Shutterstock; P199: encrier/Istock; P204: pio3/Shutterstock.

# Index

VIKING

UK | USA | Canada | Ireland | Australia
India | New Zealand | South Africa | China

Penguin Books is part of the Penguin Random House group of companies
whose addresses can be found at global.penguinrandomhouse.com.

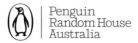

First published by Penguin Group (Australia), 2016

10 9 8 7 6 5 4 3 2 1

Cover Design by Grace West © Penguin Group (Australia)
Cover watercolour texture by Nik Merkulov/Shutterstock
Endpaper watercolour pattern by L. Kramer/Shutterstock
Text Design by Grace West © Penguin Group (Australia)
Typeset in Adobe Garamond, 10pt/14pt by Grace West
Internal illustrations by Alexia Petsinis
Colour separation by Splitting Image Colour Studio, Clayton, Victoria
Printed and bound in China by RR Donnelley Asia

National Library of Australia Cataloguing-in-Publication data is available.

ISBN: 9780670078646


penguin.com.au